Alabama Trails

To
Earle Douglas Blackburn
On your birthday 1994
Dad & Mother

*What do you suppose will satisfy the soul,
except to walk free and own no superior.*

—*Walt Whitman*

Alabama Trails

Patricia Stenger Sharpe

The University of Alabama Press

Tuscaloosa & London

The paper on which this book is printed
meets the minimum requirements of American National
Standard for Information Science-Permanence of Paper
for Printed Library Materials,
ANSI Z39.48-1984.

Library of Congress Cataloging-in-Publication Data

Sharpe, Patricia Stenger, 1948–
Alabama trails / Patricia Stenger Sharpe.
    p.   cm.
Includes index.
ISBN 0-8173-0690-0
    1. Hiking—Alabama—Guidebooks.   2.
Backpacking—Alabama—Guidebooks.   3. Trails—
Alabama—Guidebooks.   4. Alabama—Guidebooks.
I. Title.
GV199.42.A2S52   1993
796.5'1'09761—dc20   93-1640

British Library Cataloguing-in-Publication Data available

*Cartography performed by The University of Alabama Carto-
graphic Research Laboratory, Craig Remington, Supervisor,
Jon Acker, Graduate Student Assistant*

Contents

Preface

This book is an invitation and a challenge to all of us to get out and make the most of Alabama—its twenty-four state parks, eight state forests, and four national forests—and the great natural beauty Alabama has to offer the foot traveler. The park and forestry personnel in Alabama have done their best to make Alabama's trails and parks an asset to Alabamians and visitors alike, in spite of limited resources and funding. If increased interest is shown in these facilities, it may stimulate the state of Alabama and private interests to spend more of their outdoor budgets on building new trails and enhancing or maintaining current trails.

Having spent the last twelve years working in an outdoors shop, I have heard all the standard complaints about the trail-building and maintenance policies in Alabama. It is easy to be critical, especially when Alabama's facilities and budgets are compared to those of nearby states such as Tennessee, North Carolina, and Georgia. But like so many other seemingly obvious problems, there is another side. For state and local agencies to invest time and money enhancing our trails and parks, they must first see a need: More people must *request* these places. Then they must get a return on that investment: More Alabamians and visitors from other states must *use* these trails and parks.

Doctors now tell us that walking is one of the most complete forms of exercise, a practical and inexpensive way to relax your mind and body and improve your health. In making use of the trails in this book, we can not only improve ourselves but also send a message to those involved in decision making that we need and demand support of Alabama's trail system.

Acknowledgments

I wish to acknowledge all those who contributed their expertise and time to the completion of this guidebook. All the people with whom we came in contact, not only at the state and national parks but also in the state and national forest services and in the private trails sections, were gracious and helpful. While I could not always recommend certain trails I ventured upon, I have no reservations about the people I met.

I wish to thank my intrepid hiking companions: my husband, Mike, Gene Boyle, Sandra Stenger, Prissy and Larry Burrus, Barbara Malcom, Greg Messer, Joe Stenger, Margie MacGregor, Walt Williams, Tommy Cantrell, Darla and Ken Bostick, John and Lisa Montoya, Karen Newton, Brian Johnson, Keith Childers, and our friend from "down under," Ian Bilney.

Also deserving honorable mention in the patience category are: David Hogue, Alabama Forestry Commission; Danny Crownover, Lookout Mountain Trail Association; Bobby Bledsoe, Steve Jenkins, and Joy Patty of the U.S. Forest Service; my copy editor, Trinket Shaw; and the staff at The University of Alabama Press.

Lonnie Carden of Southern Trails I thank for the maps, guidance, and pithy comments on the state of our state. And, finally, my son, Jay, and my daughter, Michelle, have my sincere gratitude for reading and rereading copy, hiking some of the pits of Alabama, and eating out for three solid years.

Alabama Trails

Introduction

The purpose of this book is to provide a comprehensive listing of the trails in Alabama and to give information on their location, length, degree of difficulty, maintenance, and some of the common sights. The descriptions are brief, in order to maintain the guidebook format and to allow the volume to be easily portable. It is not meant to be read at home on the sofa or in the bathtub with vague ideas of a trip next spring. Pick it up and open to a page, put on some sturdy footgear, grab a day pack, and go. With few exceptions, everyone in the state of Alabama is within moderate driving distance of a state park, a national forest, or another site that provides day hiking for those of varying physical abilities.

This book encompasses five years of trail research, including day hiking and backpacking the actual trails and contacting the state, federal, and private agencies involved for the latest information on trail building and maintenance. Not all the trails hiked were included in this book. Some places were investigated on the off chance that they were, in fact, trails, but these were found to be no longer under maintenance or closed to public use and so were excluded. And the trails that are included are not necessarily all gems. In some cases, they were listed simply because the exclusion would have been noticed and considered an oversight (but only by those who had never hiked them). In the cases where we were less than enthusiastic about a particular trail, we have tried to be honest about its shortcomings.

The trails in this book demonstrate the enormous diversity in the state, from Little River Canyon's wildly beautiful but difficult boulder scrambling in north Alabama, to the softer, swamplike scenic strolls of the Conecuh National Forest on the southern border. All the trails are different in the demands they make on the hiker, although the majority are relatively short and moderately easy.

A massive effort was made to contact all involved public and private agencies for updates on trails, trail conditions, and future plans for trails in their jurisdictions, but as yet there is no statewide inventory, so some errors may exist. We have done our best to present accurate, current information for the use of the hiker and to warn of some of the hazards. It is also important to remember that lines on a map are not trails but depictions of trails, and a guidebook is no substitute for experience or common sense.

How This Book Is Organized

The trails in this book are divided for the sake of convenience into four areas of the state. Since most of us make our excursions on weekends, driving time becomes a concern, so we have divided the state with that in mind.

Trail markings are given where available, and trail-heads, when not marked as such, are given from a vehicle parking area.

Trail length is given as distance, not hiking time, since time varies widely from individual to individual. The time spent by a budding naturalist strolling along a given trail will differ considerably from a backpacker trying to make a long day's evening campsite. For beginners, it is always best to take a day hike or two to establish the average rate of travel before attempting a long stretch of trail. Trail length is given for a complete loop, if described as such, or for a one-way trip, if the trail begins and ends at different locations.

Degree of difficulty also varies from one person to another. I have two friends who went on the same hike, described by one as "a pretty and moderate day hike." The other has since warned others that the same trip was so horrendous that she had probably incurred genetic damage down through her grandchildren. All the trails in this book have been described as easy, moderate, or difficult. Easy trails are those that require only ordinary walking skills, demonstrate no appreciable gains or losses in elevation, and have pathways clear of obstructions. Moderate trails may require some small gains in elevation and minor scrambling over rocks, tree roots, or brush, and since the pathways are not as clear, some exertion will be necessary. Difficult trails are those that have considerable gains and losses of elevation and require advanced hiking skills and much exertion for boulder scrambling and pathway clear-

ing. These designations are all based on the average adult

in reasonable health, not professional mountaineers, triathletes, or masochists.

Maps used in this book are based on the U.S. Geological Survey (USGS) 7.5' maps that may be obtained from most trail shops or directly from the Geological Survey of Alabama, P.O. Box O, Tuscaloosa, Alabama 35486, for a modest fee. Trail shops usually carry USGS quads of local areas and popular hiking and camping areas. State road maps may be enough in some cases, but where the markings on trails are faint, USGS maps are extremely helpful. Most of the state parks will furnish maps of their facilities if asked, as will the forest service, sometimes for a small fee.

Addresses are given for private trails along with descriptions. Those wishing information on a specific national forest in Alabama should contact the district ranger or the state forest supervisor, 1765 Highland Avenue, Montgomery, Alabama 36107. For information on Alabama state parks, those interested can call 1-800-ALA-PARK, or write the Alabama Department of Conservation and Natural Resources, Division of State Parks, 64 Union Street, Montgomery, Alabama 36130.

Trail associations provide information on conditions of trails, legislation involving trails, and trips that may be open to both members and nonmembers. There are several in Alabama at this writing:

The Appalachian Trail Club of Alabama, P.O. Box 360213, Birmingham, Alabama 35236.

The Alabama Trails Association, P.O. Box 610311, Birmingham, Alabama 35261-0311.

The Lookout Mountain Trail Association, P.O. Box 1434, Gadsden, Alabama 35902.

A Word on Backcountry Manners

With more and more people journeying in fragile wilderness areas, a reminder is in order on camping etiquette. The phrase that signifies what should be our attitude in minimizing man's impact on the wild is "leave no trace." Escaping human conflict and anxiety is one of the reasons so many of us travel to the wilderness, and it is a cruel irony that we inflict so much damage on the places we go for comfort.

Fires have not yet been outlawed in parks in Alabama, as they have at sites in the Smokies and at parks in other states. Using established fire rings in established campsites diminishes the impact on the environment in high-traffic areas, since fire rings can leave scars that take years to heal. Never cut live trees for firewood; green wood rarely burns well, and it becomes a waste of forest resources. Never leave any campfires unattended. Rangers estimate that over 80 percent of the forest fires in this country are caused by people.

Carrying out the trash brought in is a matter of conscience for most hikers, but some still insist on trying to burn the unburnables, such as some foils and plastics. These should be packed out as well, even after a try at incineration, or the scraps can haunt a campsite forever.

Camp cleanups should not be done in the stream. Sending dishwater downstream for wildlife or other campers to drink is nothing more than water pollution, so carry a two-gallon collapsible water bag and do the dishwashing in camp.

A Note of Caution

Being at home in the wilderness also means understanding some of the hazards. Snakes have been seen in all parts of Alabama, and several of these snakes are considered poisonous. Rattlesnakes, cottonmouths, copperheads, and even the reclusive eastern coral snake can be found, so hikers must be alert and avoid obvious habitats if possible. Debris piles, stump holes, abandoned burrows, and rock outcroppings in brushy areas are favorites of rattlesnakes and copperheads. The cottonmouth seems to live around lowland swamps and riverine areas, while the eastern coral snake prefers moist, dense vegetation around ponds or streams.

Still in the reptile family, the American alligator is the largest reptile in North America and is found in large numbers in parts of south Alabama. It prefers fresh and brackish marshes, ponds, lakes, rivers, swamps, bayous, and large spring runoffs. While not aggressive by nature, they can be fractious during mating season in April and May, after they have emerged from hibernation. Most incidents involving harm to humans can be traced to alligators' having been fed by humans and coming to associate human beings with a food supply. This is much the same problem that has arisen over the years with the bear population in western national parks. Alligators are important to the ecology of their habitat, in that they dig deep holes, or dens, which become water holes for other animals during periods of drought.

Smaller animals, but a good deal more aggravating on a frequent basis, are the gnats, no-see-ums, ticks, chiggers, bees, wasps, and hornets that every hiker is likely to encounter at one time or another. Once again, prevention and avoidance are the keys. Assorted bug repellents will provide some measure of relief from these, and in the case of chiggers, sulfur sprinkled on the clothes seems to be a deterrent. Ticks have become an increasing problem because of their ability to spread disease. Bug repellents appear to discourage their attacks on humans, but as with chiggers, it is also best to avoid them by not sitting on woodpiles or crawling through brush. And if it is impossible to avoid contact with ticks, then frequent checking of locations ticks prefer, such as hair, waistbands, and socks, is necessary.

Noxious plants are found at some point along almost every trail in the state, the most unwelcome of these being poison ivy. Many an outing has been ruined 24 to 48 hours later by the bumps, redness, and persistent itch that may go on for days and weeks afterward. The discomfort is caused by the resin, urushiol, that adheres to the skin when plants of the genus *Rhus* are bumped or damaged. Most woodland travelers are soon able to recognize the trailing vine that branches in clusters of three oakleaf-shaped leaves. In the spring, the vine unfolds three shiny reddish leaves, and toward the end of the season, brown tendrils will branch off an inch-wide vine around trees, posts, or boulders.

One disagreement has raged for years as to the existence of poison oak in the South, and what a given three-leaved plant might be. Poison oak and poison ivy are botanically related, and one school of thought says that if it climbs, it's ivy, and if it clumps, it's oak. Whatever it might be, the best advice is to avoid contact with the plant and take special care to clean boots and equipment that have come in contact. Even the smoke of the vines burned in a campfire can be toxic. If contact is made with these plants, washing with soap and water seems to help remove the oil, and so far, over-the-counter preventatives and remedies have had only limited success. Campers should avoid all three-leaved plants if not sure of their identification. Stories abound of unfortunate campers who have rearranged the greenery for a bedroll or pulled up some ersatz toilet tissue, only to suffer for this mistake the next day.

Poison sumac is rarely seen, preferring swamps to higher ground. It resembles the familiar sumac leaf structure but has white berries. Avoid contact with the plant, since exposure causes extreme skin irritation, more serious than poison ivy or poison oak.

Another common problem that is easily circumvented is gastrointestinal distress brought on by an unsafe water supply. Avoid drinking from any water supply where there is doubt of its purity, and regard all so-called clear streams with suspicion. With more people than ever venturing into the wilderness areas, pollution of water sources is increasingly common. Waterpump-type filters, water purification tablets, carrying a supply from a potable source, or boiling will all give a measure of protection from these "bugs."

One more hazard that must be mentioned in connection with hiking in Alabama is hunting season. While the state parks do not allow hunting at any time, the national forests and trails on private land may have only limited restrictions. The best advice is to avoid these areas during hunting season, and most especially on opening weekend of a given season, since each year at least one person, and usually more, is injured or killed on opening day. Unfortunately, the fall months of hunting season are some of the most beautiful times for hiking in the state. Choosing state parks to hike in during this period is one alternative, but for most of us, this isn't always enough. If you are hiking in a national forest or on private land during the danger periods, remember to make enough noise to alert hunters to your presence, wear bright colors to be seen, and stay on recognizable hiking trails.

And, Finally, the Weather

Complaints are often made about the heat in the summers in Alabama. This situation, like bad water, is easily avoided. Don't hike in Alabama in the summer. The combination of swarming bugs, stifling heat, smothering humidity, and foliage run amok can defeat most lovers of the outdoors. But we in this state have nine months of the year that we can be outdoors without all these problems. Spring is lovely with the myriad azaleas, dogwoods, and wildflowers blooming all over the state. Fall brings crisp evenings and colorful foliage to northern Alabama, and many days throughout the winter provide bright sun and mild conditions for enjoying the backcountry with a minimum of weather gear. But if summer is the only choice, then hikers should take frequent breaks for water and should plan short, easy days with time for resting in the heat of the day.

Common sense should be the rule in any situation with potential hazards, be it wild animals, lighting, flash floods, hypothermia, rock falls, or heatstroke. Rangers, local law enforcement officers, and even trail shops can usually provide current information on the condition of trails and weather problems in a given area.

There are some beautiful places in Alabama and lessons to be learned from all the wild and free things around us. Who cannot use a few hours away from everyday routine, at an unhurried pace with time for reflection? Take this opportunity to plan a day or a weekend in the backcountry and enjoy.

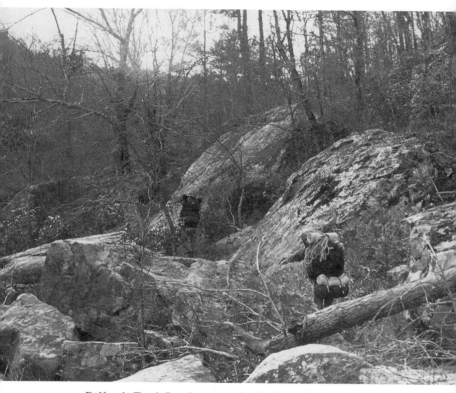

Difficult Trail Conditions in Little River Canyon, De Soto State Park (Photograph by Lonnie Carden)

Trails in North Alabama

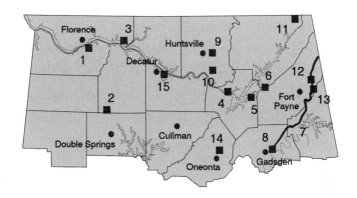

1. Muscle Shoals Reservation
2. Sipsey River Recreation Area
3. Joe Wheeler State Park
4. Honeycomb Creek Trail
5. Lake Guntersville State Park
6. Buck's Pocket State Park
7. Lookout Mountain Trail
8. Noccalula Falls Park
9. Monte Sano State Park
10. Madison County Nature Trail
11. River Mont Cave Historic Trail, Inc.
12. De Soto State Park
13. De Soto Scout Trail
14. Palisades Park
15. Point Mallard Park

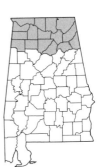

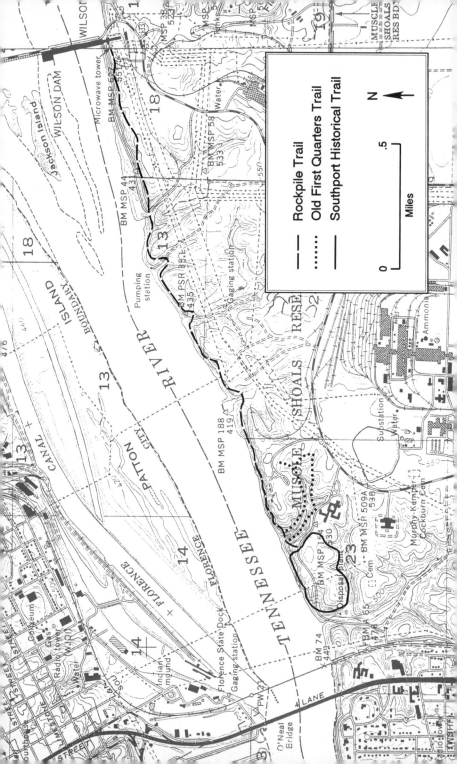

Rockpile Trail

Old First Quarters Trail

Southport Historical Trail

N

0   .5

Miles

Muscle Shoals Reservation

The Old First Quarters Small Wild Area is a facility of the Tennessee Valley Authority (TVA) Regional National Heritage Project, which works to identify and protect significant natural areas throughout TVA regions. The Small Wild Area and its trails seek to give visitors to the Muscle Shoals/Wilson Dam reservations a representation of the terrain, plants, and animals of this northwestern Alabama locale. The name First Quarters refers to the building complex that originally housed World War I military residents and later the engineers and employees who constructed Wilson Dam.

The trails are all short and moderately easy, with only occasional steep and rocky stretches, most of which have steps of one sort or another. From all appearances, the Muscle Shoals facility is the cleanest and best-maintained public TVA site in the state. The Wilson Dam Public Access facilities are not as well maintained. In fact, that area was a total disaster at the time of our visit, with the few restrooms working poorly or not at all, trash overflowing the small number of trash receptacles, and only two potable water sources for the large number of recreational vehicle and tent campers parked at the access.

The Old First Quarters Small Wild Area is located on the Muscle Shoals Reservation access road off U.S. 43 and U.S. 72 business routes, 1 mile south of the O'Neal Bridge across the Tennessee River, between the cities of Muscle Shoals and Florence.

Topo: Florence 1:24,000

Rockpile Trail

Length: 2.7 miles
Description: This trail begins 0.1 mile west of the Old First Quarters site parking area on the service road. The trail leaves the road and travels down the hill toward the overlook site through tall hop hornbeam trees. The state record hop hornbeam, or ironwood, tree resides in this area, measuring 40 inches in circumference and with a crown spread of 33 feet. After the overlook, the trail drops steeply into the ravine to cross a small wooden

NORTH
ALABAMA

11

bridge at its intersection with the Old First Quarters Trail and ascends back up along the shoreline toward the picnic pavilion.

After passing in front of the pavilion, the trail reenters the wooded shoreline of the lake and becomes a less apparent but still obvious pathway for the next mile. At approximately the 1.5-mile point, the trail enters the Wilson Dam Public Access Area, crosses the entrance road, and mounts stone steps to parallel the shore once again. The trail passes through an abandoned picnic area, passes over the huge spring that gushes with surprising force over the cliff face, and eventually exits at the power station parking area at the top of the dam.

Old First Quarters Trail

Length: 1 mile

Description: The Old First Quarters Trail traces a loop beginning at a parking area tucked between the main personnel building road turnoff and the picnic area road turnoff. A public-use trail sign exists, but it can only be seen once in the parking area. The trail is not long, but even in its short distance, it provides a sample of the varieties of plant life in the Small Wild Area. Beech, hackberry, and sweet gum trees predominate here, while the delicate maidenhair fern, the evergreen Christmas fern, the unusual walking fern, and the tree-clinging resurrection fern adorn the forest below. Leaving the parking area, the trail proceeds down man-made steps into a ravine and crosses a small wooden bridge to parallel the ravine for another 0.25 mile. The trail traverses the ravine again at an intersection with the Rockpile Trail and travels up the other side of the depression to exit the wooded area at the First Quarters site parking area. This road may be followed eastward past the original quarters foundations back to the main parking area.

Southport Historical Trail

Length: 1.3 miles

Description: This easy trail begins at the main trail parking area and makes a short loop through a series of wooded hillsides. The trail meanders around Civil War breastworks, stonework remains of the Civilian Conservation Corps period and an old graveyard dating from the period of the historic city of Southport. The trail offers good views of Pickwick Lake and provides benches near the steeper sections of the trail.

Sipsey River Recreation Area

The Bankhead National Forest has long been the site of dissension between the environmental and economic communities, but those who have hiked the Sipsey Wilderness Area, and love it, realize that it serves the interests of both sides to preserve this land for our children. The over 25,000-acre area features an unusual variety in topography, lying as it does at the intersection of the Cumberland section of the Appalachian Plateau and the Gulf Coastal Plain. This variety also exists in the vegetation to be found in the canyons and ridges of the Sipsey, where large numbers of mosses, wildflowers, grasses, and ferns flourish.

Hiking trails here exhibit this same variation, and though most are well marked and frequently traveled, all offer some physical challenge through this heavily forested and rugged country. Trails may be steep in some places and require some boulder scrambling, and most require fording creeks and the river. Hiking boots or sturdy shoes are strongly recommended. Trails in this area have few or no physical aids and range in difficulty from moderate to very strenuous, especially with a full pack.

Spring with its short-lived wildflowers and autumn with its colorful hardwoods may be the best seasons of the year. Winter, when the trees are stripped of leaves, allows the hiker to enjoy the wildness of the scenery, along with the occasional snow flurry or ice sculpture on the canyon walls. So, basically, that leaves summer for the snakes and ticks (ticks are very prolific throughout the Sipsey River area).

Although water may be available near many of the trails for most months of the year, it must be treated to be drinkable, or a supply must be carried in by the hiker. Campsite locations are unrestricted, with permits needed only during hunting season (October–April). Camping on

NORTH ALABAMA

13

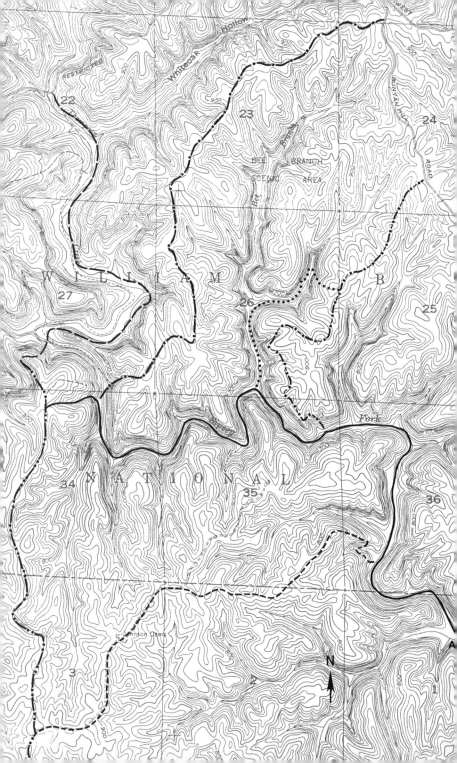

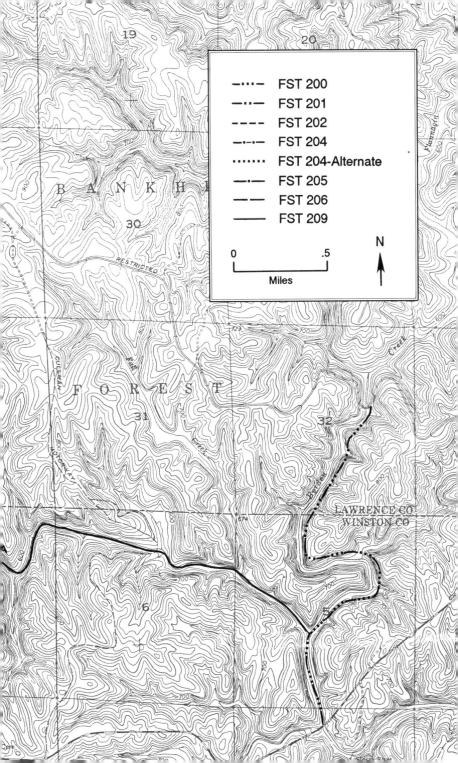

or near the banks of streams inside the canyons is discouraged, since flash flooding is always a possibility. In this high-usage area, many campsites have already been established; overnight campers should use these campsites and fire rings rather than damaging another site. Rangers in the Sipsey Wilderness Area also encourage hikers to register at trailheads for safety and for usage computations. Parking is ample at most trailheads, but vandalism has been a problem in the past at some sites. No trailhead facilities such as drinking water or restrooms exist.

Bankhead National Forest is located in Lawrence and Winston counties, with Cranal Road (County [CO] 60) serving as a southern boundary for the Sipsey Wilderness Area and Double Springs on U.S. 278 being the closest town to the area. Maps are available from the U.S. Forest Service and from some of the ranger stations for a small fee. These used in conjunction with the U.S. Geological Survey maps should provide the most accurate information on the area.

Topo: Bee Branch 1:24,000

FST 200 or Borden Creek Trail

Length: 2.7 miles

Description: This trail begins under the highway bridge at the Sipsey River Recreation Area on Cranal Road (CO 60) and moves north upstream along the Sipsey River. This trail falls into the moderately strenuous category, with stream crossings (some on logs and some on stepping-stones or just mud patches) and a few boulder-threading and deadfall-jumping exercises.

The first 0.5 mile of the trail follows the riverbank to where Borden Creek empties into the Sipsey River. At this point, the hiker may ford Borden Creek and follow Forest Service Trail (FST) 209 or may follow Borden Creek to the northeast. From this point and for the next mile, the trail narrows and crosses several small streams as it follows a horseshoe-shaped path through a canyon lined with hickory trees and tall birches. One of these streams, approximately 0.5 mile from the ford, tumbles out of a cool, green, miniature canyon, inviting a short stop and pulling the camera out of the pack.

For the next mile after the trail turns north again, it

climbs the bank of the creek, and huge rock walls over-shadow the trail, which becomes increasing rocky. At one point, the trail weaves through huge boulders and seems to disappear. A trail marker points to a large crack in the rocks where the trail then emerges on the other side of the boulders 30 feet away. It is a very narrow tunnel, so packs will have to be removed to negotiate the passage. In the winter, ice can build along the trail and passageway and can make travel very hazardous. The trail comes out of the canyon where Borden Creek widens and crosses under Forest Service (FS) 224. Parking is available here but only for two or three cars.

FST 201

Length: 2.5 miles
Description: This trail starts at the parking area of Cranal Road (CO 60) approximately 4 miles west of the Sipsey River Recreation Area. The first 0.5 mile of the trail runs parallel to or on the closed logging road from the parking area. At this point, the trail forks to FST 202 or climbs north through an area of dogwoods, pines, and oaks. Frequent deadfalls from a past tornado make this trail a moderate hike, although the terrain is fairly level until the last mile. The trail tops a ridgeline and forks east and steeply downhill along a small runoff to intersect with FST 209 or to continue along the side of the ridge until it ends at FST 206, where Thompson Creek and Quillan Creek join to form the Sipsey River.

FST 202 or Johnson Cemetery Trail

Length: 2.9 miles
Description: This moderate trail begins at the fork of FST 201, approximately 0.5 mile from the parking area at Cranal Road (CO 60). Like FST 201, this terrain is the higher forestland of the wilderness area, much different from the wet canyons that characterize the river bottoms.

The trail follows the old logging road to Johnson Cemetery, which inters some turn-of-the-century residents of the county. From this point for the next 1.5 miles, the trail winds along the ridge through large stands of hardwoods, with deadfalls and poison ivy the only annoy-

NORTH ALABAMA

ances. The trail begins to drop steeply 0.25 mile from the Sipsey River and continues down to ford the river and join FST 209.

FST 204

Length: 2.4 miles (plus 2-mile hike in along the road)

Description: This easy trail begins on the northeast side of the wilderness area off FS 224 (Bunyan Hill Road). Since the closing of FS 224 between the Borden Creek and Thompson Creek parking areas, an additional 2-mile walk up the road is required to get to FST 204. This closing was necessary to take some of the casual day-use traffic off the Bee Branch Canyon area and allow some of the signs of overuse to heal.

After the hike in along the road, a small clearing and a forest service signpost mark the entrance to the trail. The trail climbs gently from the former parking area through large oaks and poplars for almost 1.5 miles. At the trail marker, the more obvious trail (FST 204-Alternate) turns right and continues into the canyon. The less apparent FST 204 proper continues straight for another 0.5 mile through the hardwoods, staying on top of the ridgeline. The last 0.4 mile drops rather steeply into the canyon and intersects with FST 209 on the banks of the Sipsey River.

FST 204-Alternate or Bee Branch Trail

Length: 2.3 miles (plus 2-mile hike in along closed road)

Description: This may be the most familiar trail in the wilderness for most people and, for that reason, the most abused. The trail begins at the same spot as FST 204, but at the intersection and marker post 1.5 miles into the trail, this alternate bears right. At this point, the trail winds down to the edge of the Bee Branch Scenic Area and begins the 400-foot descent into the canyon itself. This is a moderately strenuous hike in and out and may be hazardous when wet or frozen. Unfortunately, the canyon has always been a favorite destination for less responsible day hikers, and it is always possible to find a good deal of trash along the trail and in the cavelike overhangs in the canyon.

The canyon has been sculpted over the millennia by Bee Branch, which currently takes a 90-foot plunge at the head of the canyon. Numerous small offshoots of the trail can take the hiker farther into the head of the canyon to the branch or to any of the small side canyons and their streams nearby. Ironically, for those who find the ice in the canyon hazardous, winter is one of the most beautiful times to be there. The lack of foliage allows the rock formations to be appreciated, and the ice formations that line the canyon walls and crack like rifle shots when breaking are splendid.

Inside the canyon, several obvious pathways lead along the stream and past numerous previously used campsites. The main trail follows the stream past huge boulders and towering canyon walls all the way to its intersection with the Sipsey River and FST 209.

FST 205

Length: 3.2 miles

Description: This easy hike starts on the north side of the wilderness area off FS 224 (Bunyan Hill Road). The trail, which tops the ridgeline for its entire length at some of the highest elevations in the wilderness area, presents no real hazards, although some deadfalls create a nuisance. After wandering south through a nearly untouched forest of oak, poplar, hemlock, and hickory trees, some of the oldest growth in Alabama, the trail drops from the ridge to intersect with FS 209.

FST 206 or Thompson Creek Trail

Length: 2.5 miles

Description: This trail begins at a parking area off FS 208 (Northwest Road) where the road crosses Thompson Creek. The first mile follows the shallow creek through a gently rolling forest of poplars and oaks. The creek bottom is wide, and except for a shallow stream crossing and several deadfalls, the hiking is moderately easy through this area. The trail then climbs gently for 0.5 mile, while the walls of the canyon become increasingly steep and the trail becomes rockier. Boulder formations and cavelike ledges loom over the trail, and the stream cross-

NORTH ALABAMA

19

ings become steep. The last 0.5 mile drops back to creekside, and the trail ends at its junction with FST 201.

FST 209 or Sipsey Fork Trail

Length: 7 miles

Description: Despite its moderately strenuous hiking, this is the longest and perhaps most interesting of all the trails in the Sipsey Wilderness Area—especially for those who like wildflowers. Bee Branch is the only other place in the wilderness area that rivals this trail for color and variety. Trillium, dwarf wild iris, showy orchis, foamflower, violet, aster, and royal catchfly are just a few found trailside along the Sipsey River in the spring. The trail begins at the Borden Creek ford on FST 200, 0.5 mile from the Sipsey River Recreation Area. The first 3 miles past the ford are as level as walking along a stream can be, with no particular hazards except for the usual numerous deadfalls. At the first 0.5-mile point, Fall Creek cascades 30 feet over a ledge to a pool, which makes a perfect rest stop or even a quick shower stop. Several other small streams are crossed along this pathway, some being easier to negotiate than others. At about the 3-mile point, FST 202 (Johnson Cemetery Trail) intersects with FST 209. A mile or so farther, this trail reaches its juncture with FST 204, and 0.5 mile onward finds the hiker at the mouth of Bee Branch Canyon. For the next 2 miles, numerous campsites may be seen along the banks of the Sipsey River, attesting to this trail's popularity. The last mile finds the river narrowing and brings the hiker to another ford. After crossing the river, the trail grunts up the canyon wall along a steep and rocky little stream to exit the canyon and intersect with FST 201.

Joe Wheeler State Park

Joe Wheeler State Park is a 2,550-acre area featuring an 18-hole championship golf course, a 134-slip marina, and convention facilities for up to 500 guests. One of Alabama's fine resorts, this state park perches on the shores of Wheeler Reservoir and offers to its visitors a full range of activities that revolve around the water, including

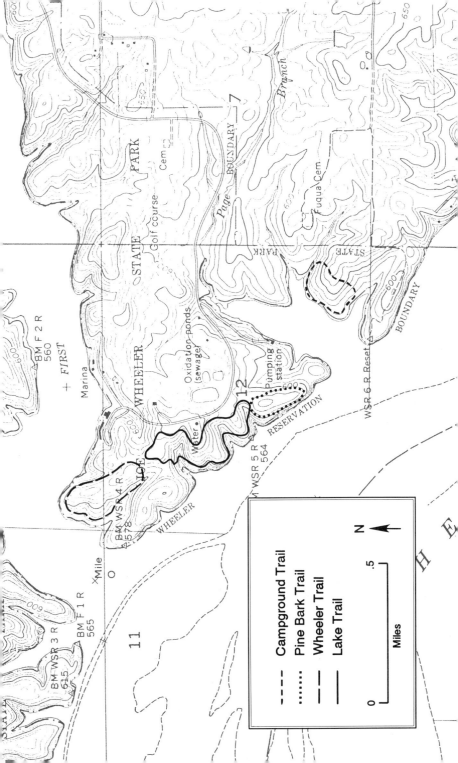

boat rentals, boat launching, swimming beaches, and fishing along the miles of shoreline.

The trails in Joe Wheeler State Park are not long or difficult, but trail markings are few and the paths sometimes dim and overgrown. Visitors to the park will find the typical north Alabama flora: tall pines mingled with oaks, maples, and colorful dogwood and cherry trees. Wildlife flourishes here at all times of the year, and watchers in the woods will see squirrels, red and gray foxes, shrews, raccoons, and opossums, depending on the time of day.

The main facility of Joe Wheeler State Park is located 2 miles west of Rogersville, off Alabama (AL) 72. The other areas of the state park include Wheeler Dam off AL 101 and the Elk River fishing facility 15 miles west of Athens. The area is open from dawn to dusk year-round, with fees for recreational vehicle and primitive camping sites but free for day use.

Topo: Rogersville 1:24,000

Campground Trail

Length: 0.5 mile
Description: Campground Trail makes a short loop at the edge of the primitive campground. No entrance sign marks the trail, but it begins across a small wooden footbridge and has orange blazes on some of the trees. After passing over the bridge, the trail mounts a hill through huge trailing vines and tulip poplars. Near the top, the path swings west and begins to drop toward the Tennessee River to follow the shoreline for 0.25 mile and return to the footbridge. Since the trail can be very mushy where it comes close to the water, footing can be hazardous.

Pine Bark Trail

Length: 0.5 mile
Description: This well-marked and well-traveled trail loops around a heavily wooded area near the day-use area. The trail can begin at either the shelter 3 parking circle or near the service road to the tennis and basketball courts. Red blazes point the way through hazelnut trees, honeysuckle vines, and buckeyes. This trail connects with Lake

Trail by a small wooden footbridge at the northern end of the trail.

Wheeler Trail

Length: 1 mile
Description: This loop also receives a good deal of traffic because of its proximity to the lodge. The trail leaves the lodge and follows blue blazes down to First Creek to move along the shoreline for a short distance. It then climbs along a small draw to crest a hill, passes near the tennis courts, and returns to the lodge area.

Lake Trail

Length: 1.3 miles
Description: This loop, the longest trail in the park, begins and ends off the service road near the lodge tennis courts. The trail is much the same as others in the park but has better views along the lakeshore. The pathway, blazed intermittently in yellow, is heavily wooded and overgrown in places but is not difficult to follow. Since it connects with Pine Bark Trail by a small bridge and almost connects with Wheeler Trail via the service road, a longer hike can be made by combining the three paths.

Honeycomb Creek Trail

Honeycomb Creek Trail forms part of the Honeycomb Creek Public Use Area on Guntersville Reservoir. This area, set aside for the people of Alabama by the Tennessee Valley Authority (TVA), includes campsites with picnic tables, water and electrical hookups, playgrounds, boat launching ramps, bathhouses, and a beach area. In spite of a pavilion, the campground mysteriously specifies no picnicking, but that may be in reference to the small number of campsites available.

The currently maintained section of the trail—the first 1.7 miles—offers no special challenge to the hiker and takes a pretty lakeside stroll through pines, hickories, and a few elms. The waterfowl that use the area are plentiful and a joy to observe even without the pleasant shoreline

NORTH ALABAMA

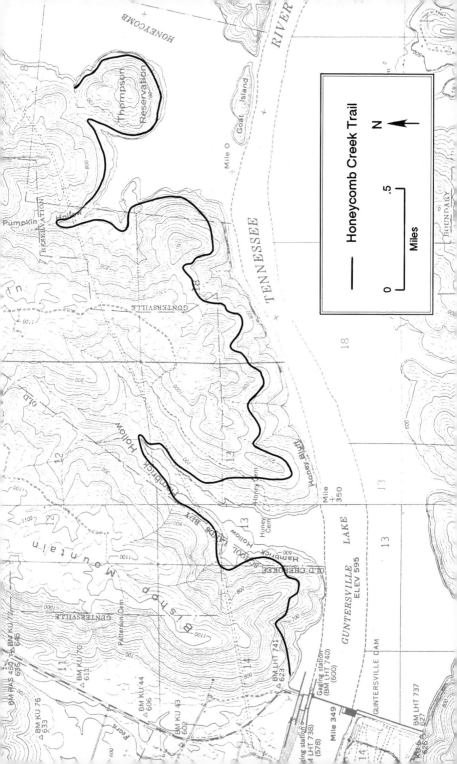

scenery. The trail crosses several small ravines, but all have wooden bridges and, in some cases, handrails.

The Honeycomb Creek Public Use Area is located off U.S. 431, approximately 11 miles north of the city of Guntersville, and is open from 6 A.M. to 10 P.M. daily. There is no entrance fee, but there are fees for camping. For more information contact TVA, Norris, Tennessee 37828.

Topos: Guntersville Dam, Mount Carmel 1:24,000

Honeycomb Creek Trail

Length: 6.7 miles

Description: The trailhead is located at the far southern end of the campground in a small parking area with a sign. The first 1.7 miles, maintained by TVA, makes an easy hike for the whole family, if used as a walk-in and return on the same route. It follows the lakeshore closely around the Thompson Reservation point, through a draw known as Pumpkin Hollow and into the undeveloped Honeycomb Creek Small Wild Area. From this point onward for the next 5 miles, the trail is unmaintained and obscured by growth. Hugging the shoreline along the Tennessee River channel, where the banks become rugged and rocky, the trail climbs the hillside and continues 150 to 250 feet above the water. Skilled hikers with a map, compass, and perhaps a machete for the overgrowth, will eventually find themselves at Honey Cemetery and an old jeep trail. The trail then circles Hambrick Hollow for a mile or so and begins to drop off the hill to Guntersville Dam. Trash, a problem in so many public-use areas, is prevalent for the first and last mile of the trail.

Lake Guntersville State Park

Lake Guntersville State Park, another one of the splendid resorts in Alabama's state park system, provides almost any facility that a vacationing couple or an entire convention could ask for. Accommodations within this 5,559-acre park may be found in lakeside cottages, in chalets situated on the 500-foot bluff near the main lodge, or in the huge recreational vehicle and tent campground.

NORTH
ALABAMA

25

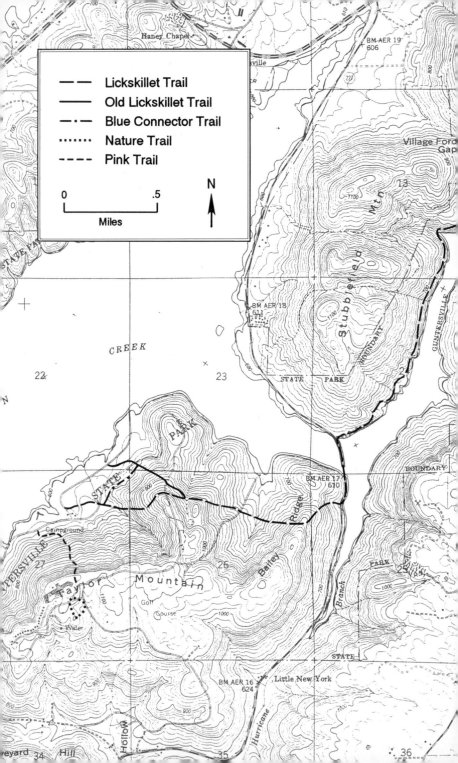

Legend

- — — Lickskillet Trail
- ——— Old Lickskillet Trail
- —·—· Blue Connector Trail
- ········· Nature Trail
- – – – Pink Trail

N

0   .5

Miles

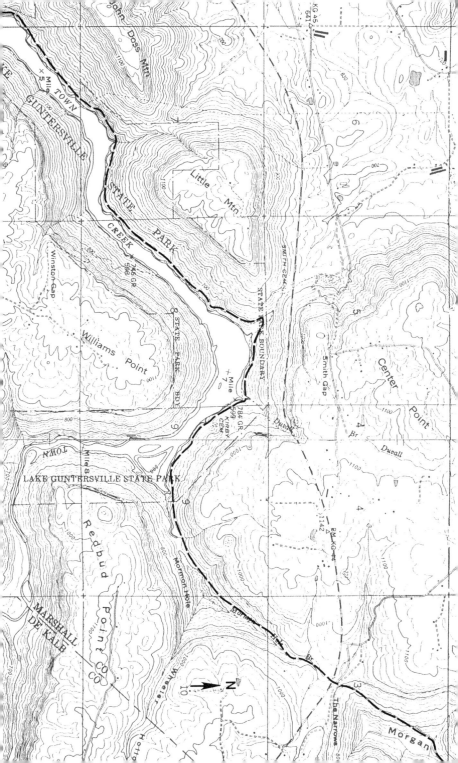

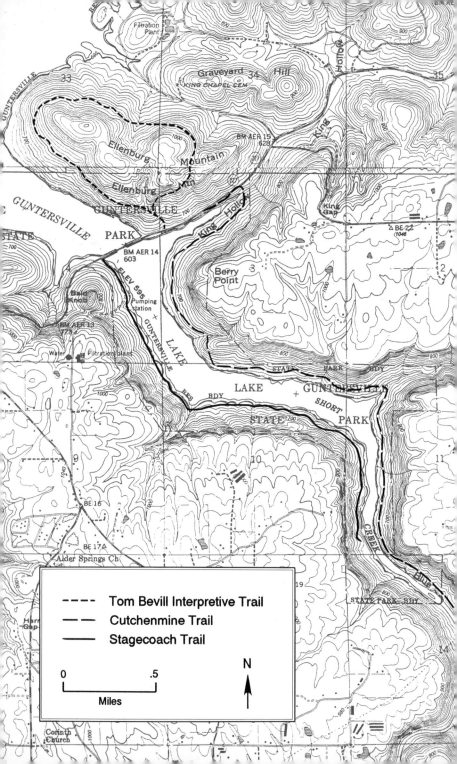

Tom Bevill Interpretive Trail

Cutchenmine Trail

Stagecoach Trail

0   .5

Miles

N

From the 18-hole golf course on top of Taylor Mountain to boat rentals at the beach, this state park has something for everyone.

Marshall County recreation has been centered around the Tennessee River and Lake Guntersville since the Tennessee Valley Authority (TVA) built Guntersville Dam in 1929 and donated 1,700 acres of shoreline to the state for a park. Besides being renowned for its bass fishing, this park is also a wildlife preserve, with a unique combination of lake and mountain environments. Deer, turkeys, groundhogs, opossums, hawks, and foxes number just a few of the local inhabitants who have been joined by a newer group of occupants—the eagles. These birds had become more and more rare in Alabama, but in the last few years, a group has made a resurgence in the park.

Hiking here has as much diversity as the ecology. Trails range in difficulty, from a very easy 20-minute stroll suitable for the whole family, to a moderately strenuous 12-mile lakeside hike, to a 1-mile straight up (or straight down) "killer grunt."

Other facilities include the lodge restaurant and gift shop, tennis courts, swimming pool, golf course pro shop, basketball and volleyball courts, boat-launching ramps, camp store, and picnic pavilions. No fees are required for day use of the park, which is open from dawn to 10:00 P.M. Lake Guntersville State Park is located off Alabama (AL) 227, 6 miles northeast of the city of Guntersville.

Topos: Columbus City, Albertville, Grove Oak 1:24,000

Lickskillet Trail

Length: 3 miles to Town Creek fishing camp
12 miles to Buck's Pocket State Park

Description: Lickskillet Trail begins opposite the campground store on the park's service road. The portion up to Town Creek fishing camp should be considered moderate, while the portion from Town Creek fishing camp to Morgan Cove Road should be considered difficult.

The trail climbs the side of Taylor Mountain through tall oaks, poplars, and pines. This very clear path appears to get a good deal of traffic, although as it nears the road, a number of other trace trails develop. Several colors of

NORTH
ALABAMA

blazes mark the trail, but orange seems to predominate. After climbing for 1.5 miles, the trail crosses the skyline drive service road and enters a large group of pines to meander toward the lake. The track drops through a small runoff ravine, climbs, and then comes steeply down off Bailey Ridge to intersect with AL 227.

Crossing the highway bridge over Town Creek, the trail enters the fishing camp, passes the camp store, and for a short distance follows an old jeep track along the shore. The track dims considerably in the next 4 miles and becomes little more than a fishing path along the lakeshore through brambles and overgrowth. At the 5-mile point past the fishing camp, the shoreline of the lake turns sharply south, and the trail leaves the shore to move eastward toward the depression known as Mormon Hole. The trail skirts the depression and follows the small creek known as Mormon Hole Branch toward AL 227. A compass is a must here, since this section is almost impassable due to blackberry and dewberry brambles and the large amount of trail overgrowth. This area, which could be very pretty, would make a great scout project for a cleanup campaign.

At AL 227, the trail travels down Morgan Cove Road (the turnoff is 30 yards south of the trail) to join the Primitive Campground Road and Trail in Buck's Pocket State Park (see next section). The trail leaves Morgan Cove Road 0.1 mile from the Morgan Cove parking area and travels east. The trail is obscured by a large number of all-terrain vehicle tracks, but by bearing east, the hiker can easily pick up the trail and follow it up South Sauty Creek to the state park.

Old Lickskillet Trail and Blue Connector Trail

Length: 0.4 mile

Description: Old Lickskillet Trail originates 0.5 mile north of the beginning of Lickskillet Trail on the same service road to the golf course. No markers show the start of the trail, but a clearing in the trees is still apparent. Past the opening, the trail is clear from the amount of use it has had in the past. The trail ascends the side of Taylor Mountain for a short distance to intersect again with the service road. The short Blue Connector Trail joins Old

NORTH
ALABAMA

Lickskillet Trail to Lickskillet Trail, both of which have blue and orange blazes and are considered moderate.

Nature Trail

Length: 0.5 mile
Description: This loop starts at the base of the lodge parking lot next to the tennis courts. The trail, a project of Boy Scout Troop 171, is a wide, easy walkway through pines and hickories.

Pink Trail

Length: 1 mile
Description: The signs at both ends of this trail read "steep and difficult." Its designers apparently dropped a huge steel ball from the top of the hill; where it rolled straight down, they put pink blazes on trees but have since allowed erosion to take care of trail maintenance. The trail originates behind the playground next to the lodge and parachutes down the side of Taylor Mountain to end across from the country store at the campground entrance. If looking for the trail from the campground side below, the sign can be difficult to see, but it is opposite the store along the side of the service road. (If planning to try to do this trail from the store up to the lodge, the hiker may need ice-climbing crampons.)

Tom Bevill Interpretive Trail

Length: 3 miles
Description: The first 100 yards of this nature trail are the hardest, but if that steep stretch can be survived, the rest of the trail is easy, fairly level, and a real pleasure. The trail begins across the road from the park manager's office, near the AL 227 bridge over Short Creek. An interpretive booklet can be obtained from the park naturalist's office, but at this writing, many of the numbered site signs were missing. This loop allows the hiker to see many ongoing forest ecological processes, such as the symbiotic relationship of algae and fungus in lichens, the effects of wind, ice, and fire on trees, and the damage the southern pine beetle wreaks on the forest. Sassafras,

NORTH
ALABAMA

pines, chestnut oaks, muscadine vines, and a large grove of locust trees salute the hiker on this trip. Several of the nature sites relate to an old homestead, a freshwater spring, and the settlers and Creek Indians who lived here in the 1800s.

Cutchenmine Trail

Length: 4 miles

Description: Cutchenmine Trail derives its name from a late 1800s miner who built a flume to Short Creek to get his coal to civilization. This relatively easy trail is fairly level as well, but it does require more care in stepping over rocks along the shoreline and across small ravines created by the erosion of the banks of Short Creek. The trail originates just east of the park manager's office on AL 227 and is bracketed by the lakeshore and the highway for a short distance before turning south to ford a small creek. The trail continues along the shoreline, retracing the pathways Cutchen used and traveling through hardwoods and pines. The trail, which ends near a set of rapids where Short Creek empties into the lake, returns along the same path.

Stagecoach Trail

Length: 2.5 miles

Description: Since this trail is relatively new to the park, it is not yet marked well or traveled extensively. It is not a difficult trail, in that it is relatively level and follows the contours of the lakeshore, but it is considered moderate because of the overgrowth, lack of markings, and dampness. The trail starts on the west side of the AL 227 bridge near the park manager's office. At this writing, no sign marked the entrance, but the trailhead can be found between the lake shoreline and the utility company road 20 feet away. The trail goes and returns along the same pathway.

Buck's Pocket State Park

Straddling the DeKalb–Jackson County lines, Buck's Pocket State Park ranks as one of the park system's most

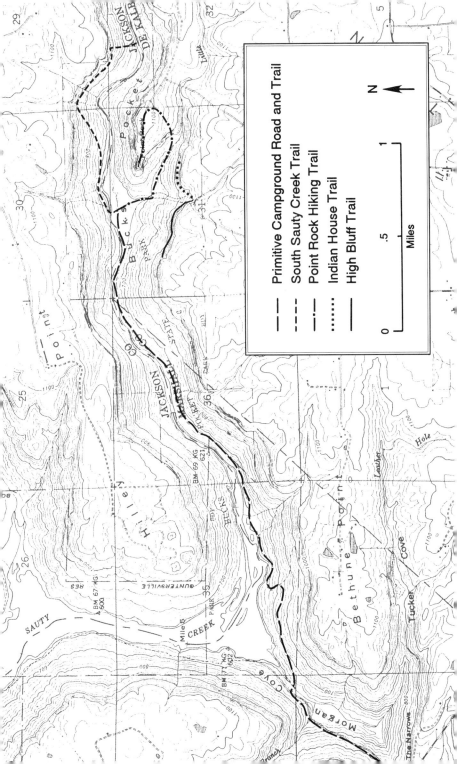

Primitive Campground Road and Trail
South Sauty Creek Trail
Point Rock Hiking Trail
Indian House Trail
High Bluff Trail

N

Miles

0   .5   1

picturesque facilities. From the park's observation over-look at the 1,100-foot-high Point Rock, to the base of the canyon and South Sauty Creek, the scenery is superb. Legends of the derivation of the park's name range from the tradition of the Cherokee Indians' hunting buck deer in the pockets of the canyon, to the abundance of the cupped husks found on certain types of acorns, or buckeyes.

The trails of Buck's Pocket vary widely in difficulty, as well as length, from boulder scrambling on Point Rock Trail, to an easy walk on the Primitive Campground Trail. The rugged 2,000-acre facility has wheelchair-accessible restrooms, a playground, picnic areas, and overnight campsites with hookups. Backpacking is required to get into the most primitive sites, a nice touch for those who wish to get away from recreational vehicles and day-use traffic.

The park is located 10 miles northwest of Fyffe off Alabama 75 and 2 miles north of Grove Oak off County 50. While there are no charges for day use, there is a fee for overnight camping. A trail guide and information sheet can be obtained at park headquarters.

Topo: Grove Oak 1:24,000

Primitive Campground Road and Trail

Length: 2 miles to camping area
8 miles to Town Creek fishing camp

Description: This trail leads to the only planned primitive camping area at Buck's Pocket State Park. The trail provides easy walking, since it follows an old access road along South Sauty Creek to Morgan Cove, a backwa-ter of Lake Guntersville. To reach the road, turn right at the campground entrance and drive to the bottom of the canyon. The parking area will be on the left side of this road.

The first mile of the road gives visitors a very good look at the rock formations that line the creek and a portion of the canyon not visible from Point Rock. After the first mile, the creek gradually widens and forms the backwater for Lake Guntersville. At the 2-mile point, the trail widens, and the bank of the backwater opens into a clearing that forms the primitive campground. Facilities include a beach area for those who wish a swim in Lake

Guntersville and even a picnic table or two, which means the area will sometimes be shared by primitive campers and day users as well. This represents easy hiking for the most part, with almost no elevation gain or loss. Good access to water all along the trail figures as a mixed blessing, though; the flying insect population, which also enjoys the proximity of the water, can be a real problem at certain times of the year.

For those interested in quieter areas, a better suggestion would be to travel 2 or 3 miles farther on the same pathway and escape some of the traffic. After the clearing, the track narrows and rises off the bank of the backwater. A mile later, after crossing a small creek, the trail turns north and joins Morgan Cove Road, which may also be used as access to the trail. Unfortunately, this area experiences a great deal of traffic from all-terrain vehicles, and the foot trail is often obliterated by the large number of tracks they leave. The Primitive Campground Road and Trail ends here and becomes Lickskillet Trail and travels on through Morgan Cove to Lake Guntersville. For more information, see Lake Guntersville State Park.

South Sauty Creek Trail

Length: 2.5 miles

Description: To reach South Sauty Creek Trail, drive past the campground entrance and across the creek to the Jackson County side. The entrance to the trail lies only 50 yards past the creek but is somewhat overgrown, so it is possible to miss, at least was at the time of this writing. This trail parallels South Sauty Creek for the first 0.5 mile and is a well-marked, easy walk through rhododendrons and several species of mountain laurel and trillium. The trail then climbs the ridge in a moderate gain in elevation and descends in the next 0.5 mile to end on the banks of the creek again. This trail may provide the most opportunities for both naturalist and photographer. Plans for a primitive campground at the terminus of the trail have been discussed, but the area remains unimproved at this time.

Point Rock Hiking Trail

Length: 2 miles

Description: This trail originates on the entrance road bridge near the park headquarters and follows an old logging road dating from the 1930s. Since it also parallels Little Sauty Creek for over half the length of the trail, it presents the hiker with cascading waterfalls at some times of the year and the challenge of slippery rocks at all times of the year. The rockiness and steepness of the trail in some spots give this trail a moderate rating.

After fording the creek, the trail mounts steeply toward the cliffs to end at the tip of Point Rock, the highest peak in the park. While wildflowers bloom profusely along the creek in the spring, autumn, another favorite time of the year, finds the trees at their most colorful. Fewer leaves on the trees also make it possible to see more of the geological formations, including the Big Sink, an underground water cavern. One caution to visitors: the top of the formation known as Point Rock has no guardrails in certain spots and has a very steep and long drop-off at the edge.

Indian House Trail

Length: 0.3 mile

Description: Shortly before the entrance road drops into the canyon, Indian House Trail begins. The trailhead is well marked, and the path presents an easy stroll through a multitude of rhododendron and spectacular rock formations. The trail ends at one of these rock formations, a large overhang known as Indian House, which was used by the Cherokee. Care should be taken in and around the formations, as the rocks are often slippery.

High Bluff Trail

Length: 0.5 mile

Description: The entrance to High Bluff Trail is located at the pull-off on the DeKalb County side of the park at the top of the steep S curve. This short moderate trail winds around and through huge cliffs and rock formations and traverses a small creek. The trail ends with a view of the western portion of the canyon. While not an arduous climb, the trail necessitates careful walking around the rocky areas and through the creek crossing.

Lookout Mountain Trail

Lookout Mountain Trail is an ambitious enterprise that was begun by the former Alabama Appalachian Association and the Lookout Mountain Trail Association. Upon completion, this trail will be one of the South's longest and most scenic, stretching from Noccalula Falls in Gadsden, continuing across the northwestern corner of Georgia, and concluding some 100 miles north atop Chattanooga's Lookout Mountain at the Chickamauga National Military Park.

Hikers visiting the trail will find unusual rock formations, striking panoramic views, cascading waterfalls, some plants that are found only in this area of the state, and the small animal life that characterizes northern Alabama. Lookout Mountain, one of the southernmost peaks of the Cumberland Range, ranks as a close relative of the Great Smokies. The trail ranges from moderate hiking in the Gadsden area, to very difficult hiking deep in Little River Canyon. No facilities will be found along the trail itself, and water may not be available, so it is best that the hiker plan to be self-sufficient. Public camping facilities, water, and restrooms are available at Noccalula Falls Campground, Canyon Mouth Park Campground, and De Soto State Park. The trail is marked with white blazes similar to those along the Appalachian Trail, to which the organizers hope some day to link it.

At one time known as the J.F.K. Trail, it was nearing completion at the time of this writing, but signs and blazes are missing in some section. Lookout Mountain Trail crosses private as well as public lands, and hikers are advised to travel only on the trail through these areas to avoid friction with local landowners. Overnight camping should be restricted to public areas and campsites previously established. For those interested in further information and updated trail conditions, contact Danny Crownover, 609 South 4th Street, Gadsden, Alabama 35901.

Topos: Gadsden, Gadsden East, Keener, Leesburg,

**NORTH
ALABAMA**

37

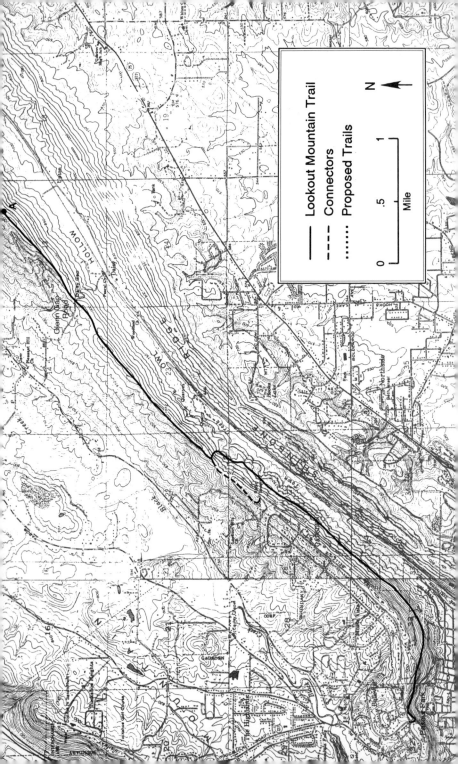

Lookout Mountain Trail
Connectors
Proposed Trails

N

0   .5   1
Mile

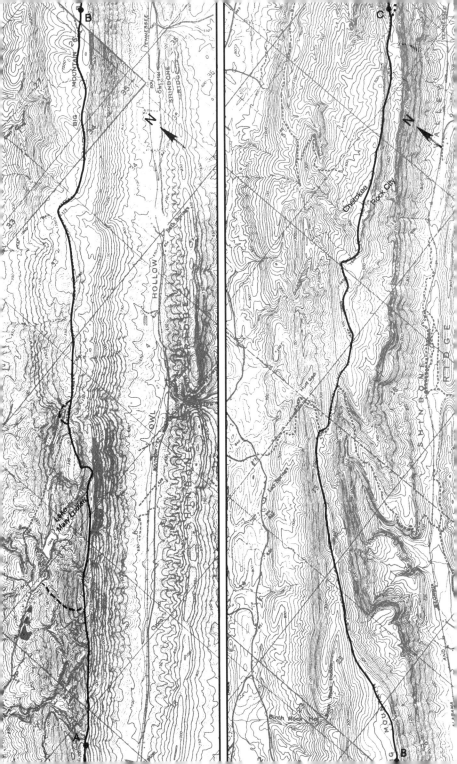

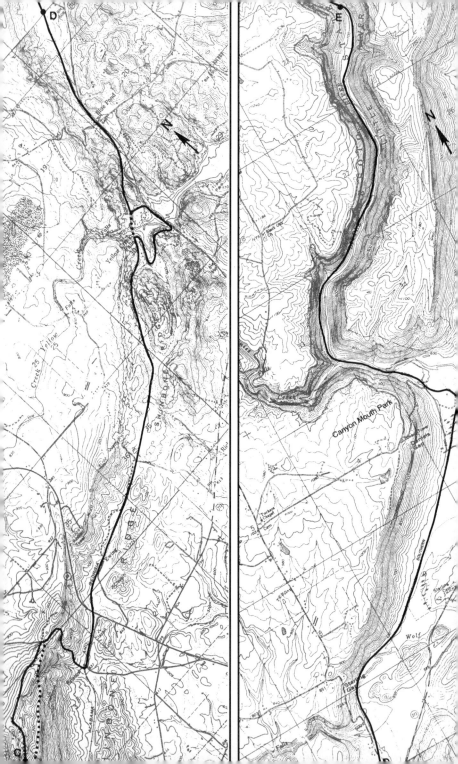

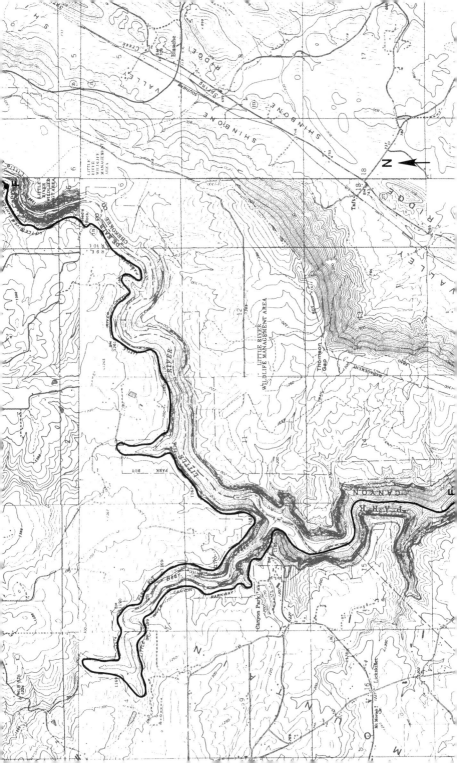

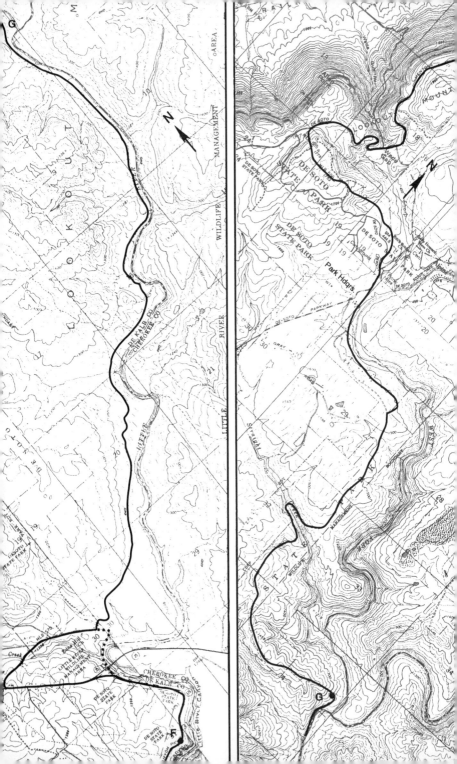

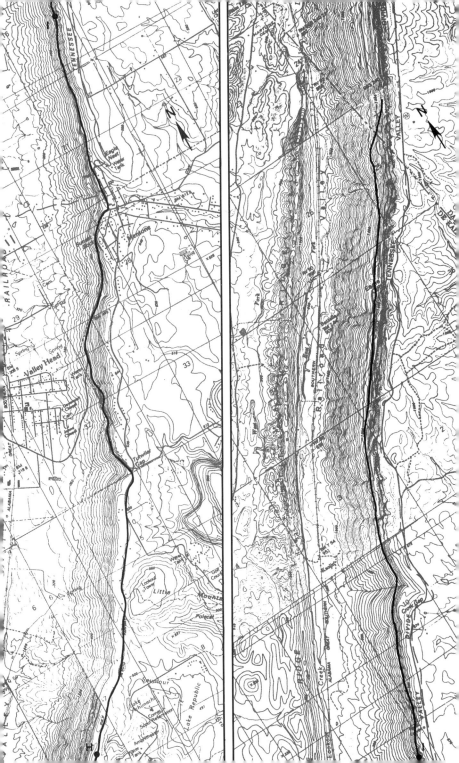

Centre, Little River, Fort Payne, Jamestown, Dugout Valley, Valley Head, Sulphur Springs 1:24,000

Paseur Park to Glenn Gap Road

Length: 5 miles

Description: Lookout Mountain Trail currently begins at Paseur Park on Highland Avenue in Gadsden near Noccalula Falls Park. At some point, the trail planners hope to connect the trail to the park itself through the Gadsden War Memorial area. Parking, but no other facilities, is available at Paseur Park. The trail crosses Highland Avenue and travels up the heavily wooded hillside to remain at an 800-foot elevation for several miles. The trail intersects Overlook Drive at the 1-mile mark, giving another entry point to the trail.

Hikers can also access the trail from the south end of South Belmont Drive off Lay Springs Road, along a 0.25-mile connector called Cablevision Trail. Parking is not allowed at this access point without prior approval of nearby landowners, and cars left blocking the road to the radio and cable towers will be towed away. The trail rises as it nears Daisy Gap, offering the hiker views of Town Creed and nearby Shinbone Ridge before it crosses Glenn Gap Road.

Glenn Gap Road to Cherokee Rock City

Length: 12.5 miles

Description: After leaving Glenn Gap Road, the trail rises slightly and follows the edge of the ridge for 2 miles, passing near Lake Mary Louise. This area is posted against trespassing, so hikers should not stray from the path toward the lake. The trail climbs very steeply for 0.25 mile and reaches a formation known as Sand Rock House, a popular camping spot with views of the valley and a nearby spring. Lookout Mountain Trail rejoins the old jeep trail for 5 miles of moderately easy hiking to Huff Gap. Unpaved Huff Gap Road intersects the footpath at approximately the 10-mile point and provides another entrance or exit for the trail. Huff Gap was a late 1800s settlement, and old cellars, foundations, and wells may still be seen. Hikers

NORTH
ALABAMA

44

should take care to avoid falling into one of these remaining overgrown structures.

Because Cherokee Rock City is a well-known rock-climbing and bouldering spot, weekends can produce a traffic jam of climbers, campers, and visitors. These enormous rock formations provide spectacular views—several states may be seen on a clear day—and its ledges, small caves, natural bridges, and chimneylike projections make it an intriguing place to camp or spend a lunch break. Trash represents the only problem here, with a liberal mixture of broken glass, paper wrappers, and Alabama's substitute for planted roadside wildflowers, the aluminum can.

Cherokee Rock City to Yellow Creek Falls

Length: 7 miles

Description: Lookout Mountain Trail follows the gravel road along the top of the ridge for 2 miles, where it reaches a four-way intersection of old roads and then drops south off the top of the ridge along a firebreak road. Viewing sites intermittently along the roadside offer panoramas of nearby Weiss Reservoir and the Coosa River Valley. Plans for this section of the trail in the future include bringing the trail down the ridgeline nearer Cherokee Rock Village, but at this time, it stays on top of the road. At the bottom of the hill, the trail joins the old Tennessee, Alabama, and Georgia Railroad bed, which provides relatively easy hiking for several miles. The bed still has tracks for the next mile, but the railroad has plans to remove these.

At the 4-mile point, Lookout Mountain Trail crosses Alabama (AL) 68 and passes the old Ewing Mill. The pathway stays relatively flat for the next 3 miles to the falls where Yellow Creek cascades off Lookout Mountain, another popular rock-climbing location. Crossing the railroad bridge is not the safest thing to do, owing to the distance between timbers; we suggest that the hiker leave the trail along the road at the base of the bridge and walk out to the highway to cross Yellow Creek on the AL 273 bridge.

Yellow Creek Falls to Canyon Mouth Park

Length: 6 miles

Description: Crossing Yellow Creek, the trail picks up the first paved road on the left and follows it back to the railroad bed. Skirting the community of Blue Pond, the trail travels through Starling Gap toward Little River, designated as an Alabama Wild and Scenic River. This section of the pathway moves along the railroad bed for its entire length to Canyon Mouth Park at the south end of Little River Canyon. The trail leaves the railroad on County (CO) 275 into Canyon Mouth Park, a private campground with limited facilities.

Canyon Mouth Park to Canyon Park

Length: 7 miles

Description: Upon entering Little River Canyon, the deepest gorge east of the Mississippi, the trail becomes a part of De Soto State Park. Floods and landslides over a period of several years have made the pathway almost impassable. But since the park service has no funds for trail building or maintenance at this time, and since volunteers are scarce, work continues only intermittently on this very difficult section. For more information, see De Soto State Park, Little River Canyon Trail. Lookout Mountain Trail leaves the banks of Little River at the old chairlift and follows an old jeep track, a steep and rutted journey climbing 600 feet in elevation, to exit the canyon near Eberhart Point Park.

Canyon Park to AL 35

Length: 17 miles

Description: The next 17 miles of Lookout Mountain Trail follow Little River Canyon Parkway (AL 176), an easy walk on a paved surface past some of the most-photographed overlooks in Alabama. While no camping is allowed in Canyon Park, several of the overlooks provide picnic tables. The first 6 miles of the parkway snake around Bear Creek Canyon, an extension of Little River Canyon, and pass Grace's High Falls, the highest waterfall in Alabama. Farther along the parkway and directly across from Eberhart Point, near the place where hikers exit Little River Canyon, rises Crow's Point, which offers one of the best views of Little River Canyon from its highest point of 600 feet.

Umbrella Rock, close to the 10-mile point in this section, presents an unusual formation in the middle of the parkway, with a boulder "village" nearby. The parkway leaves the edge of the canyon as it becomes shallower and soon intersects with AL 35.

Note that while the walking is easy in this section you must watch out for vehicles. This road is narrow and winding and visibility in many stretches is extremely limited.

AL 35 to De Soto State Park Headquarters

Length: 12 miles

Description: This section starts at the Hill Memorial Bridge over Little River on AL 35. The proposed trail will cross Yellow Creek and intersect with a logging road 0.2 mile north. However, the current route heads north on AL 35 and turns right on the first dirt road, passing Edna Hill Church, an early "circuit rider" church and the southern terminus of De Soto Scout Trail. From this point and for the next 6 miles north, the trail follows De Soto Scout Trail (see that chapter).

At approximately mile 6, Lookout Mountain Trail breaks from De Soto Scout Trail along a jeep track and turns up the ridgeline away from Little River. From this point on to De Soto State Park, few signs exist on Lookout Mountain Trail, and several sections remain under construction at this time. The trail continues on the jeep track for 4 miles, crossing an old Civilian Conservation Corps bridge over Straight Creek and running along the park service road in the cabin area. The marked pathway follows the Rhododendron Trails to the park headquarters.

De Soto State Park Headquarters to Mentone

Length: 13 miles

Description: From the park headquarters, Lookout Mountain Trail coincides with the Rhododendron Trails through the park to the De Soto Parkway exit. Once on

NORTH
ALABAMA

the De Soto Parkway, the trail currently follows the parkway to the Mentone community. In the past, the pathway traced the De Soto Scout Trail all the way past the community of Alpine and Lake Howard to Comer Scout Reservation; hikers may want to choose this route instead of the parkway.

Mentone to Alabama State Line

Length: Approximately 12 miles

Description: This portion of Lookout Mountain Trail, now under construction, may be largely completed within the next year. The trail will parallel the Tennessee Valley Divide and AL 157 all the way to Cloudland Canyon State Park in Georgia and into the National Military Park in Chattanooga, Tennessee.

Noccalula Falls Park

Etowah County's most historic park and campground nestles among the rock formations and hollows near Noccalula Falls. The name refers to a legendary Indian princess who leapt to her death from the top of the 90-foot falls rather than marry a brave who had been chosen for her by her father but whom she did not love. This attraction, atop a mountain on the west side of Gadsden, is owned by that city and is maintained as a joint venture by the Gadsden Jaycees and the Parks and Recreation Department.

The park includes a pioneer log village, tourist facilities and a museum, a replica train ride, playgrounds, a picnic area, and a huge botanical garden containing over 25,000 azaleas. The moderately easy nature trail in the park area has markers and physical aids for hikers, but care should be taken in the wetter and rockier areas. The facility plays host to a large area craft show in early October and an art show in May each year. Brochures and a trail map can be obtained at the entrance to the park.

The park, on Noccalula Road off Interstate 59 and U.S. 431, charges a fee for admission and additional fees for camping and recreational vehicle hookups. For more

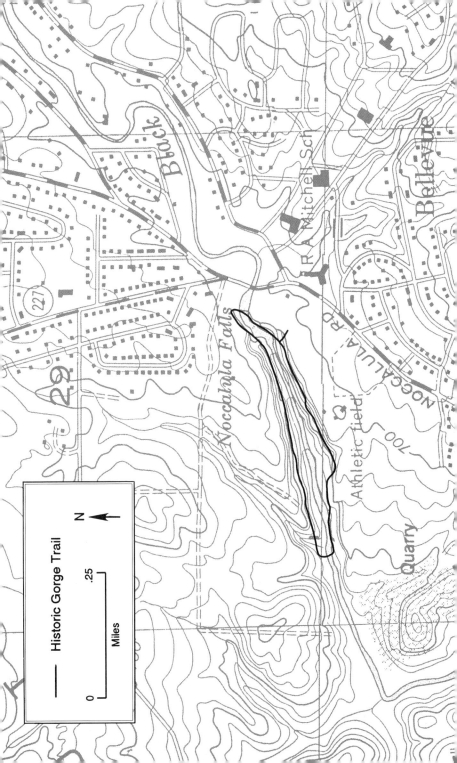

information, contact Noccalula Falls Park, P.O. Box 267, Gadsden, Alabama 35999.

Topo: Gadsden 1:24,000

Historic Gorge Trail

Length: 1.5 miles

Description: Yellow blazes on the trees mark the way as the Historic Gorge Trail encircles the 500-foot-wide gorge chiseled by Black Creek as it cascades down Lookout Mountain and over Noccalula Falls. In the gorge's earliest days, the falls were located at Chalybeate Springs; however, the gorge has since lengthened to over 3,000 feet. The trail begins near the entrance to the park and enters the gorge on the metal steps. Originally, wooden steps installed in the 1870s led to a dance platform under the falls, and the small spring that provided drinking water for the dancers can still be seen.

Moving out from the falls and looking northwest, the hiker spots Keener Cave, a reported Civil War hideout and moonshining location. Within the next 0.25 mile, a large crack or joint appears in the gorge and spouts a small waterfall through the rock. The ruins of a nearby aboriginal fort can be seen as a large "room" behind a boulder near the crack.

Close to where Cascade Creek enters Black Creek lies an abandoned mine channel, as well as the remains of a dam where a natural swimming hole was built. The rocks and the walkway throughout this area are slick and footing hazardous, so care should be taken. After passing Chalybeate Springs, a pre–Civil War health resort, the trail crosses a suspended bridge and circumnavigates an 1890s pumphouse. For the next 0.25 mile, the trail wanders through a mountain laurel and hydrangea thicket, until it joins a roadbed built years ago by the city and completes its loop back to the falls.

Monte Sano State Park

Perched atop Monte Sano Mountain, this 2,140-acre state park offers outdoor experiences near the heart of Huntsville. Monte Sano State Park resulted from a project

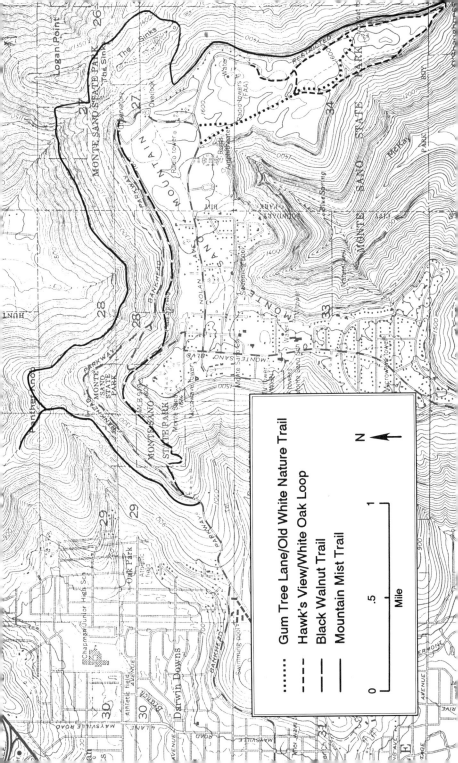

Gum Tree Lane/Old White Nature Trail

Hawk's View/White Oak Loop

Black Walnut Trail

Mountain Mist Trail

N

Mile

0   .5   1

of the mid-1930s Civilian Conservation Corps (CCC), which was responsible for building the park's stone cottages and even the cottage furniture. Today the park contains hiking trails, picnic areas and pavilions, recreational vehicle and primitive campsites, playgrounds, cabins, an amphitheater, a planetarium, and a country store.

Large oaks, poplars, sycamores, and pines shelter small mammals and shade the hiker on walks along the trails. The park's mountaintop location and easy access to a large population center make it a popular day and weekend getaway.

Monte Sano State Park, located at the eastern city boundary of Huntsville off U.S. 431 and Monte Sano Boulevard, is open daily from 8 A.M. to sunset, with no fees for day-use facilities.

Topos: Huntsville, Meridianville 1:24,000

Gum Tree Lane / Old White Nature Trail

Length: 1.5 miles

Description: The easy Old White Nature Trail originates at the hiker's parking lot off the main service road near the park headquarters. The pathway traces an old jeep trail up the side of the mountain past now-abandoned nature stations, an open-air theater, and small streams. It connects with Gum Tree Lane (blue blazes) and traverses a clearing on top of the mountain near the lookout tower to join the logging road.

Hawk's View / White Oak Loop

Length: 3 miles

Description: Beginning at the end of the park service road near cabin 14, this easy trail offers the best view of surrounding Madison County. The first 0.5 mile traces a logging road toward a lookout tower, but then the trail leaves the road, following red blazes, and moves south along the top of the ridge toward panoramic O'Shaughnessy Point. Past the point, the trail hugs the rim northward for another 0.25 mile before dropping off the mountaintop for a short distance. Tall pines and wind-blown oaks line the walkway all the way back to its terminus at White Oak Trail. White Oak Trail (white blazes)

climbs up the mountainside back to the logging road to the end of the service road.

Black Walnut Trail

Length: 2 miles

Description: Black Walnut Trail starts on the park service road near the observatory and moves down Monte Sano Mountain, paralleling Bankhead Parkway. This easy trail, marked with yellow blazes, drops slowly off the mountain, with pine, walnut, and tall oak trees lining the pathway. The trail ends on the road but can be combined with Mountain Mist Trail and Gum Tree Lane for a much longer loop of approximately 9 miles.

Mountain Mist Trail

Length: 5.5 miles

Description: Mountain Mist Trail, the park's longest and most challenging trail, ranks as a moderate walk because of the downed trees and the up-and-down character of the pathway. The trail begins on an old logging road off the service road entrance to the north end of the park. With orange blazes to guide the hiker, the trail wanders through the heavily wooded hillside for a mile toward Panther Knob. Leaving that lookout point, the trail travels again along the side of the mountain for another mile toward a low-lying area known as the Sinks and then passes the quarry where the stone was removed by the CCC to build the park's cabins. Crossing the bottomland, the trail rises toward the cabins, where a connector trail allows the hiker to exit or to enter from the park's main service road between cottages 6 and 7.

The next 2 miles of the trail hover just below the brow of Monte Sano Mountain and move through an area of deadfalls, junked cars, and trash. This portion of the trail has suffered a tornado and several ice storms, which account for the large number of downed trees, and the junked cars may be an effort on the part of park officials to enshrine this art form as the Alabama state sculpture. But the presence of enormous amounts of broken glass on the trail argues not only for heavier penalties for trashing state lands but also for the arming of park rangers. The trail,

**NORTH
ALABAMA**

53

easily followed if not particularly attractive, eventually ascends the mountain to end at O'Shaughnessy Point.

Madison County Nature Trail

Madison County Nature Trail circles a 17-acre lake atop Green Mountain and provides a noteworthy natural experience for visitors and a sanctuary for north Alabama plants and wildlife. Since the site was donated to the county and the trail opened in 1976, officials' hard work and reverence for beauty have made this park a quiet and lovely place for people and animals.

Spring, the most appealing season for the park, displays a vast array of plants and flowering shrubs. However, autumn, when hardwood species begin to turn colors and the weather becomes cooler, proves equally attractive. Over 300 species of trees, shrubs, and plants flourish in the park, with many labeled at the site and many identified in the main pavilion at educational displays.

The park opens daily all year, except Christmas, with the gates locked at sunset. The park, charging a small fee for entrance, features a pioneer cabin, a small chapel, a covered bridge, picnic tables, a pavilion, restrooms, and a visitor's center. Most of the park facilities and a good portion of the trail rate as suitable for all members of the family and for handicapped visitors as well. The park lies just off South Shawdee and Bailey Cove roads on the south side of Huntsville near U.S. 231. For more information, contact Madison County Nature Trail, 5000 Nature Trail, Huntsville, Alabama 35803.

Topo: Farley 1:24,000

Main Trail

Length: 1.5 miles

Description: The trail starts at the main pavilion on top of 1,335-foot-high Green Mountain and heads toward the lake through azaleas and other native plants. Having crossed the dam and tuneled through a 90-foot-long covered bridge, a replica of one that once spanned the Flint River, the pathway traverses an old homestead site, with a circa-1810 cabin and farm implements. Two side

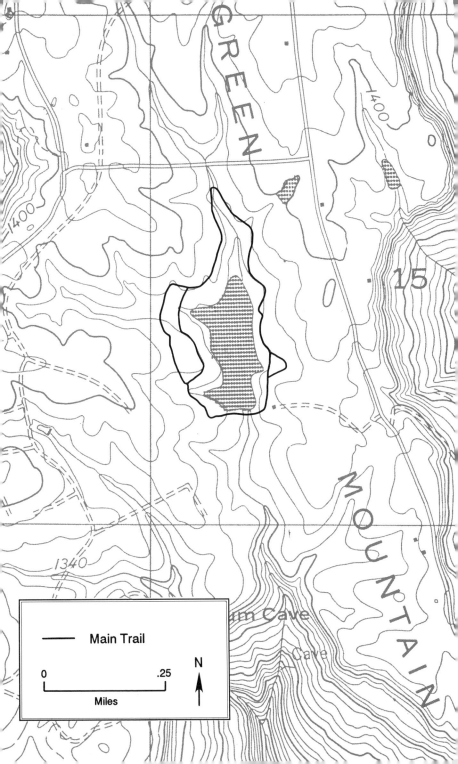

GREEN

1400

1400

1400

. 15

MOUNTAIN

1340

am Cave

Cave

Main Trail

0   .25   N

Miles

trails originate here: School Trail and Braille Trail, which provides plaques to aid the blind in the identification of plants and natural features in the park.

For the next 0.5 mile, the trail wanders away from the lakeshore through drier upland woods, fording two small streams on wooden bridges. The trail then reapproaches the shoreline, passes a small A-frame chapel, and crosses a 100-foot-long suspension bridge to complete its loop back at the main pavilion.

River Mont Cave Historic Trail, Inc.

Opened for public use in 1967, River Mont Cave Historic Trail, Inc., provides a look at parts of Alabama's past, from the era of primitive man through the Civil War to the Gay Nineties. The trail has been approved as a historic trail by the National Council of the Boy Scouts of America, which awards a medal and patch to any scout who successfully completes the journey. River Mont Cave Historic Trail exhibits more diversity in terrain than any other trail in the state, traveling from the banks of a river, along city streets, over hills and pastures, and onto rural highways.

Camping is available near the start of the trail and atop Summerhouse Mountain with prior arrangement. Hikers can find restrooms and fresh water at Russell Cave National Monument but no food or camping facilities. Water is scarce along the trail, though, so hikers are advised to bring a supply.

The trail currently presents some problems in routing as a result of new construction along the Tennessee River. Even though much of the trail covers paved surface, it still has a moderate rating because of the very steep and overgrown stretch of trail that climbs and traverses Summerhouse Mountain.

Although no charge is levied for use of the trail per se, a small fee is asked from those who wish to obtain the Boy Scouts commemorative patch and medal. However, permission is required for access to the trail and the private property involved. Current information on the state of the trail and permission for use can be requested from Bobby Hill, Troop 65, 711 Diamond Avenue, Bridgeport, Ala-

NORTH
ALABAMA

56

bama 35740 (205-495-3941). For scout troops and larger hiking groups, a 10-day notice for use of the facilities is suggested.

Topos: Bridgeport, Doran 1:24,000

River Mont Cave Historic Trail, Inc.

Length: 12 miles

Description: The trail originates in the city of Bridgeport near the same location from which the Union Army ferried supplies between Chattanooga and Bridgeport during the Civil War. Signs along the major thoroughfares in the city direct the hiker toward the railroad bridge along the banks of the Tennessee River. A small parking area exists under the bridge, but no signs are present at this time. For those interested in the trail, however, a representative from Troop 65 can arrange to meet the group with parking and current trail information.

Beginning at the bridge, the trail mounts Battery Hill toward a residential area along Olcott Avenue, giving the hiker a chance to enjoy a panoramic view of the Tennessee River. It continues along the avenue, passing restored homes of the 1890s and, farther on, the railroad yard along Hudson Avenue. Watch for signs for River Mont trail on power poles beside the route.

The trail crosses U.S. 72 along 10th Street and moves into another residential area, where, at the end of a small side street, it skirts a wooded area for 0.5 mile and joins a county road. Down the road a mile, the trail intersects County 74 and jogs north for 100 yards to follow the gravel road up the side of Summerhouse Mountain. After a few hundred yards, it exits the road to the left (south) and climbs the mountain, a very steep ascent that produces a noteworthy view from Summer Bluff.

River Mont trail sweeps along the paved and gravel roads on top of the mountain to a residence called Summerhouse Hill. A small sign beyond the driveway of this house shows the route the trail takes back into the woods. The trail soon becomes a dimmer trace, with white and red markings for the next mile to Split Rock, a large boulder formation, and on to Split Rock Bluff. The view from Split Rock Bluff encompasses the next few miles of the trail, all the way to Russell Cave National Monument. Passing Split

**NORTH
ALABAMA**

57

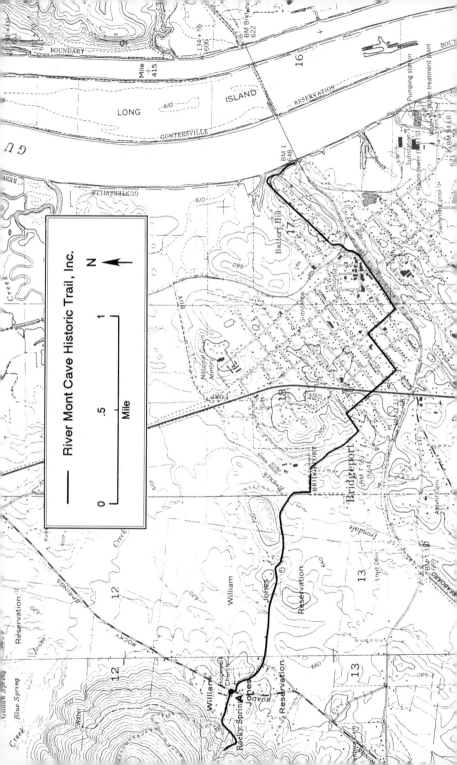

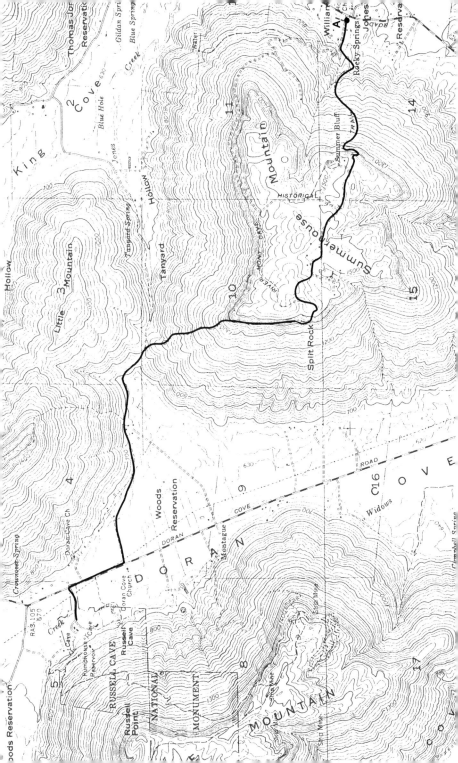

Rock, the path teeters on the brow of the hill for a short distance, begins to drop from the mountain, and then descends acutely, partially along a jeep trace, to end at the edge of Doran Cove Road, which in turn leads to Russell Cave National Monument.

De Soto State Park

De Soto State Park encompasses some of the most spectacular scenery in the southeastern United States. The hiking in some areas is quite challenging but is well worth the time and effort spent. Developed in the mid-1930s as a Civilian Conservation Corps project, the park represents part of Alabama's outstanding park resort system and offers complete facilities for both conventions and vacationers—chalets and cabins, as well as the lodge, and a large recreational vehicle and primitive camping area, with a country store, laundry area, and information center nearby. The day-use area includes a large number of picnic tables, a pavilion, and short interpretive nature trail.

The park comprises 4,990 acres within a 35-mile-long area from De Soto Falls to the mouth of Little River Canyon, with an elevation of 1,835 feet at its highest point. Little River Canyon creates one of Alabama's most unusual and beautiful natural attractions. Called the Grand Canyon of the South, this ranks as the largest gorge east of the Mississippi, and a plan is currently being proposed to place the canyon under the protection of the national park system. Little River also maintains status as the only river that originates and flows almost totally on top of a mountain.

Spring may be the ultimate time to travel through the park, when it abounds not only in azaleas, mountain laurels, rhododendrons, pines, and hardwoods, but also in sprightly wildflowers, including several rare species. Wild-flower buffs can find species of trillium and lady's slipper in the spring and Indian pipe in the fall. Throughout the year, visitors to this area can not only hike in superb and relatively unspoiled surroundings or fish in Little River, but they can also visit Sequoia Caverns and Manitou Cave in neighboring communities and, during the winter, ski

Alabama's only slopes in nearby Mentone. De Soto State Park lies 8 miles northeast of Fort Payne on County 89. The year-round park opens at dawn and closes at dusk, charging fees only for overnight camping.

Topos: Dugout Valley, Fort Payne, Jamestown, Valley Head, Little River 1:24,000

Rhododendron and Hiking Trails

Length: 20 miles

Description: This set of trails forms a network throughout the park. Signs and identification markers delineate most of the trails, although some appeared to be missing at this writing. These trails have no particular start or finish but meander through some of the most beautiful scenery in the park. The sections that adjoin De Soto Scout Trail, known as Rhododendron Trails, are picturesque but are also much more challenging, in that they move along the river itself and require some scrambling over rocks that are wet most times of the year. Sturdy shoes or good boots are a must for these sections. Other segments move through and around the campgrounds, picnic areas, lodge, and cabins, providing arresting contrasts between boulders and glades, hardwoods and blooming shrubs, and waterfalls and small streams. These gentler pathways through the park, as opposed to those through the canyon, are mostly level or gradually sloping, with footbridges and handrails at the trickier points, and so remain accessible to all the family.

Azalea Cascade Interpretive Trail

Length: 0.7 mile

Description: The park's interpretive nature trail makes an easy 45-minute loop, beginning at a three-car parking area near the country store. Through a self-guiding hiking brochure, available for a small fee at the information center, the trail showcases the trees and plants of the park, as well as some interesting rock formations. Since portions of the trail are very rocky and may be wet, particularly where it crosses Laurel Creek before the creek empties into the West Fork of the Little River, good shoes will help. Other physical aids in the form

NORTH ALABAMA

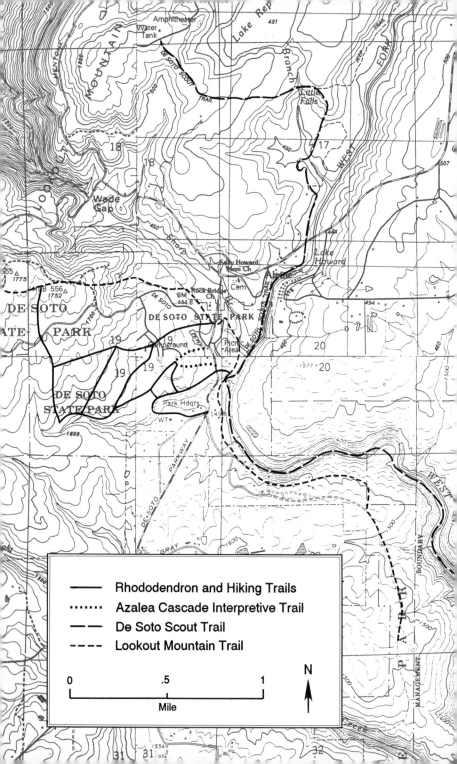

Legend

— Rhododendron and Hiking Trails
···· Azalea Cascade Interpretive Trail
– – De Soto Scout Trail
---- Lookout Mountain Trail

0   .5   1

Mile

N

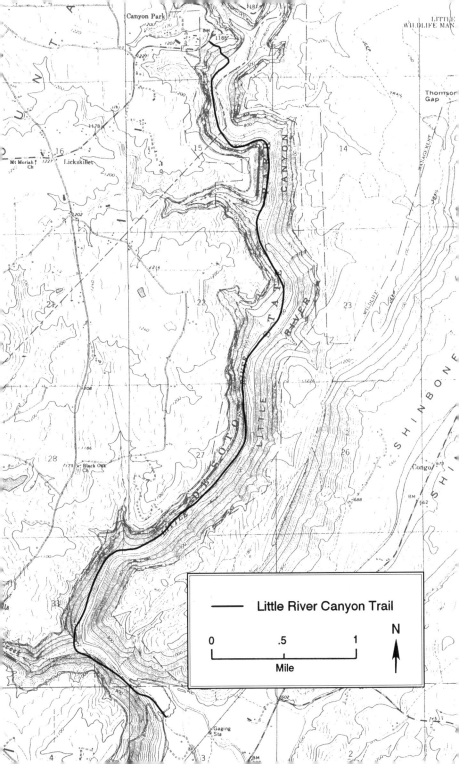

Little River Canyon Trail

0   .5   1

Mile

N

of footbridges and handrails exist on parts of the trail, so this would be a suitable trek for those family members who might find the rest of the canyon too strenuous. The well-marked trail ends back at the park's service road, where a short walk north brings the traveler back to the original parking area.

Little River Canyon Trail

Length: 7 miles

Description: This trail is not for the beginning hiker: sturdy, well-fitted hiking shoes or boots and some amount of conditioning is recommended for this strenuous journey. Visitors normally hike the trail from Canyon Park south to Canyon Mouth Park because of the steep grade at the north end; those who hike through Little River Canyon on Lookout Mountain Trail from Gadsden will have to gain the elevation from south to north.

At this writing, it is an understatement to say the north end of the canyon is in very poor shape. A scout troop of our acquaintance describes it as a "death march." Apparently, they did not enjoy the wonders of hopping over boulders, clambering over stumps, and tripping lightly through vast patches of poison ivy. The north entrance to the trail can be found along Alabama 176, approximately 50 yards north of where the chairlift for Canyon Park enters the canyon. Hikers will find a boat-launch sign some 25 feet down this trail. Do not panic. For those without boats, this also serves as the hiker's access. This entrance is very steep and eroded, but after a 0.25-mile trip, the base of the chairlift and the river can be seen.

The trail originates just south of the base of the chairlift, but it may take some brush beating to locate it. The first 2 miles of the trail are plagued by deadfalls, landslides, and huge logjams, as reminders of recent high-water periods. Although several private groups are planning cleanups in the future, only an optimist would expect to travel through this end of the canyon quickly without a machete or a chainsaw. Part of our group resorted to hiking along the riverbank on the gravel bars, but that is not possible throughout the entire canyon and is certainly not advisable in wet weather, when flash flooding in the narrow confines of the canyon is always a possibility.

NORTH
ALABAMA

64

Many of the large boulder areas feature alternate pathways around the rock, but these are usually steep and may be overgrown. Chinquapin Creek enters the canyon 1.5 miles from the bottom of the chairlift, as the trail ascends the wall for a short distance.

Soon after the 2-mile point, the path levels out, and Powell Trail drops from the rim, creating an emergency exit from the canyon. The next 2 miles present an avenue of house-size boulders, small streams to ford, and tall pines, as the river begins to widen. Less than a mile from the end of the trail, Johnnys Creek enters the canyon. The bridge that once spanned the water is gone, but because of the large rocks in the creek, fording it is merely a matter of stepping across, although this does become a problem in wet weather. The trail exits the canyon at Canyon Mouth Campground, a private area where overnight parking and camping can be arranged.

Overnight camping is not allowed in the canyon, although exceptions for cleanup crews and trail-building groups have been made. Hikers should take the ruggedness and difficulty of the terrain into account when planning a trip, so as to allow enough time to exit before nightfall. The trip length is estimated at from 7 to 9 hours without long rest stops.

De Soto Scout Trail

The De Soto Scout Trail originated with the Sequoyah District of the Choccolocco Council of the Boy Scouts of America (BSA), and many scout troops since have donated time and effort to maintain it. Scout participation may also contribute to its reputation as one of the busiest trails in the state. Yellow markings on trees blaze the trail and, in places, indicate mileposts and emergency exits.

Benefiting from the nearby facilities of De Soto State Park and Comer Scout Reservation, this DeKalb County trail winds through outstanding scenery but not without a good deal of effort. The terrain varies, but the stretch along the banks of Little River proves extremely rugged and boulder strewn, and for this reason, the entire trail

NORTH
ALABAMA

65

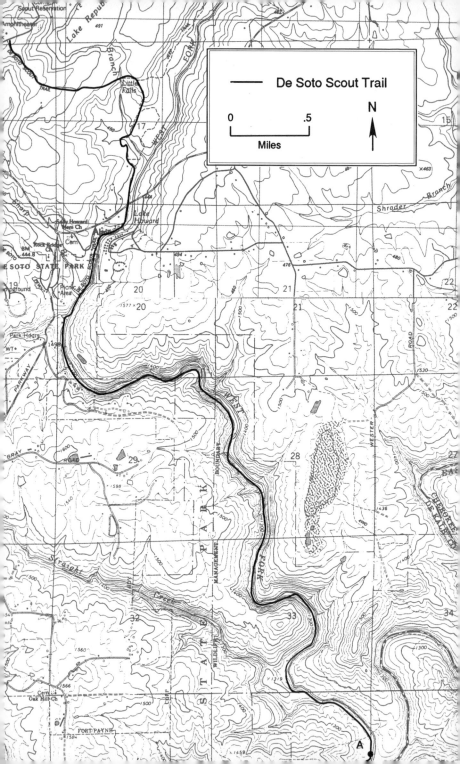

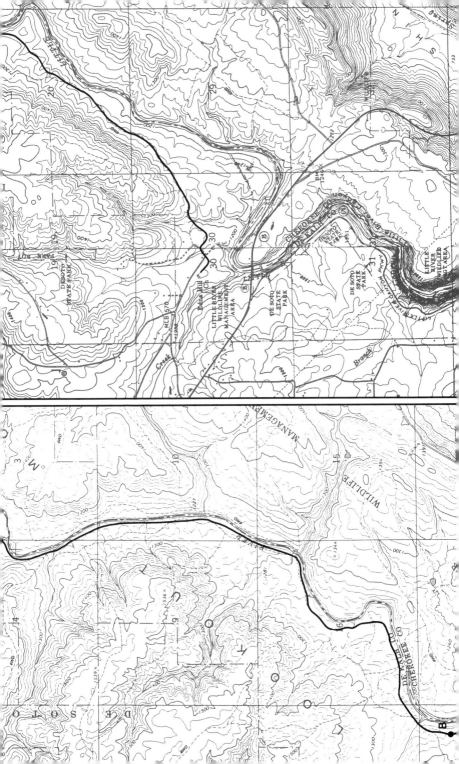

should be considered difficult. This difficulty of parts of the trail and the total length of the trail should make overnight camping a consideration. Those planning to hike or camp here should come prepared with suitable equipment and sturdy hiking boots, if at all possible. Spring, with its mountain laurels, rhododendrons, and wildflowers in bloom, and autumn, with its exuberant foliage and cooler temperatures, represent the best times to visit (however, the trail is closed from November 1 to December 31 for deer-hunting season).

The trail joins not only Lookout Mountain Trail but also the Rhododendron Trails of De Soto State Park (see maps of previous chapter). Comer Scout Reservation, the northern terminus of the trail, lies 4 miles south of Mentone on the De Soto Parkway in DeKalb County. No fees are charged for use of the trail, although those wishing to use Comer Scout Reservation as a campsite or to obtain a copy of the scout brochure and map should check with the Choccolocco Council Headquarters, BSA, P.O. Box 4549, Blue Mountain Station, Anniston, Alabama 36204, or the camp ranger, Comer Scout Reservation, Route 1, Mentone, Alabama 35984. Maps of De Soto Scout Trail are also available at the De Soto State Park Headquarters.

Topos: Fort Payne, Jamestown, Valley Head 1:24,000

De Soto Scout Trail

Length: 16 miles

Description: Beginning at the northern end, at a service road on Comer Scout Reservation, the trail follows the road across Little Falls and south toward Lake Howard in the tiny community of Alpine. After passing the dam that forms Lake Howard, it skirts a 1930s Civilian Conservation Corps shelter, one of the many stone structures erected throughout De Soto State Park. Once inside the state park, the pathway closely traces the course of the West Fork of Little River and in several spots intersects the park's Rhododendron and Hiking Trails. This beautiful segment of the hike, with its small, rocky waterfalls and towering canyon walls, also presents a very rugged side; the path is overgrown in a number of places, and the combination of briers and boulders makes travel laborious. The trail is well marked, although in any case, it would be difficult to stray without ropes and ascenders for scaling the steep canyon walls.

Exit routes have been provided at several locations in the canyon in the event of sudden high-water conditions, and prudent overnight campers and even day hikers should take note of these locations. In fact, visitors would be well advised to avoid camping along any stretch of the trail deep in the narrow portion of the canyon.

Near the halfway point, the west and east forks of Little River merge, and the topography opens up as the river widens slightly. Several river crossings present themselves within the next 4 miles. These fords were used by early settlers and even today make good spots to cool off in hot weather or to explore the opposite side of the river. One of these, Billy's Ford, facilitated the transport of a portion of the Cherokee Nation to the Tennessee River on their way west along the Trail of Tears.

The hike joins a jeep track 3 miles from the southern terminus, and traveling becomes easier. Some logging activity in the area makes finding the yellow blazes on trees difficult, but with a map, the hiker should soon find Edna Hill Church, the southernmost end of the trail. From the highway, Edna Hill Church stands 0.5 mile north of Alabama 35 and 0.5 mile west of the bridge over Little River.

Palisades Park

Set on a rugged mountaintop in Blount County, Palisades Park lists a variety of activities in its repertoire. Hiking, picnicking, nature study, and even rock climbing are here to be enjoyed in the county-operated facility. Showing off for visitors, sundrops, Indian pinks, wild roses, dwarf sumac, prickly pear cactus, strawberries, and muscadine vines all represent common plant life to this area. Those who venture here can even see the pioneer home of Daniel Murphree, one of the early settlers to the area, a cabin that was moved here and restored to its original condition in 1973.

Very well kept by a full-time superintendent, the park

NORTH ALABAMA

69

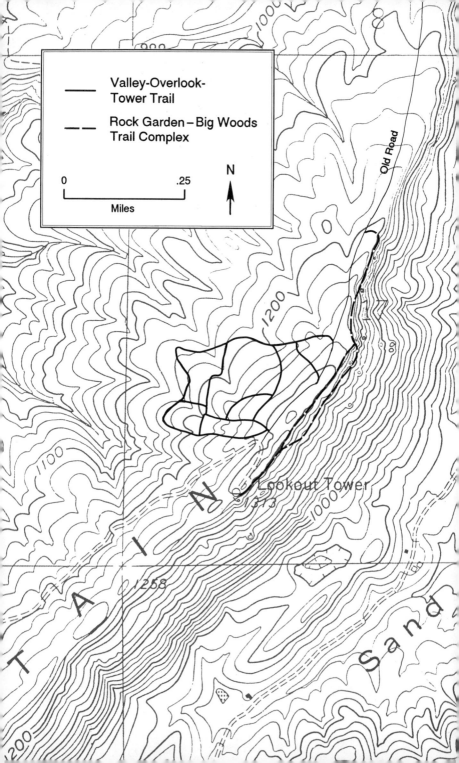

Valley-Overlook-
Tower Trail

Rock Garden – Big Woods
Trail Complex

0 .25

Miles

N

features walks that are for the most part short and in the easy category. The most obvious caution is to those who might venture too close to the edges of the rock outcroppings, lose their footings, and fall. Especially close watch should be kept on children, who find the rock formations and the old lookout tower fascinating places to play.

Since the trails all link with one another and cover a good deal of the same kind of terrain, several descriptions are combined here for the sake of simplicity. Picnic tables, shelters, playgrounds, a group lodge, restrooms, and drinking water are available. Open at no charge from 8 A.M. to 5 P.M. in the winter and until 9 P.M. in the summer, Palisades Park lies 3 miles north of Oneonta off U.S. 231 at the turnoff sign. The sign to the park may not be easily visible but is located right at the Rosa and Oneonta city boundary signs. For more information, contact the Blount County Park Board, 308 5th Avenue East, Oneonta Alabama 35121.

Topo: Oneonta 1:24,000

Valley-Overlook-Tower Trail

Length: 1.5 miles

Description: This trail network starts at the old lookout tower and offers the best scenic views in the park. The pathway northward is obvious, since countless rock climbers and those who like the more informal rock-clambering approach have scrambled around here. In this portion, where Tower Trail intersects with Overlook Trail near the picnic pavilion, rock overhangs and outcroppings of all shapes and sizes make it a popular sunning and eating spot. Overlook Trail continues along the same pathway, passing huge rock islands that appear to have broken free from the ridge to settle a few feet away. Onward 0.25 mile, the trail passes the lodge, veers away from the edge of the cliff line, and enters the woods to end at Big Woods and Old Road trails.

Valley Trail branches off the ledge walk below Tower Trail and circumnavigates the rock formations and tall pines. It parallels the rock face and, after a short distance, climbs the hill to intersect with Overlook Trail.

NORTH
ALABAMA

71

Rock Garden–Big Woods Trail Complex
(includes Old Road, Rockledge, Big Woods, Pine,
and Rock Garden trails)

Length: 2.5 miles

Description: This group of trails gives visitors the best look at the wildlife of Sand Mountain. The hiker has only to venture a few feet from the road to find ground squirrels, gray squirrels, finches, jays, and woodpeckers. Since all of these short trails connect, they can be traveled in any direction and in almost any combination. One of the prettiest hikes, an easy walk through rolling terrain and towering trees, begins on Old Road Trail near the parking area, proceeds to Rockledge and Big Woods Trail, turns to Pine Trail, and ends where Rock Garden Trail rejoins the entrance road.

Point Mallard Park

Point Mallard Park, a 750-acre complex located on the banks of the Tennessee River and owned by the city of Decatur, touts itself as a year-round facility with activities appealing to all members of the family. In addition to a full hookup campground, it offers an 18-hole golf course, a miniature golf course, an outdoor skating rink, a wave pool, athletic fields, and swimming and fishing areas.

Bird lovers will find this an especially interesting place, since many species winter here and in nearby Wheeler Wildlife Refuge. The park's namesakes, the mallard ducks, as well as Canada geese, cardinals, woodpeckers, and robins all reside in abundance, along with other representatives of the local wildlife, such as opossums, rabbits, foxes, and raccoons.

Located off Mallard Drive in southeast Decatur, the park does charge fees for camping and for most other activities but no usage fee for the trail. For more information, contact Point Mallard, 1800 Point Mallard Drive SE, Decatur, Alabama 35601.

Topo: Decatur 1:24,000

NORTH
ALABAMA

72

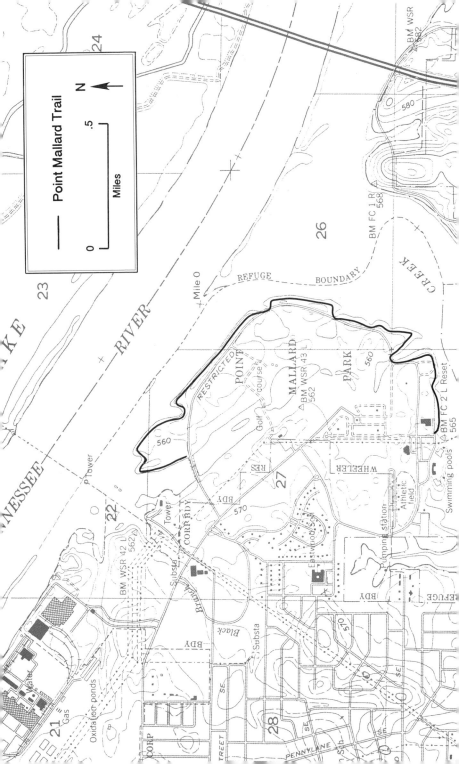

Point Mallard Trail

Length: 3 miles

Description: This trail was originally planned and built in 1972 for hiking and bicycling. Now nature walkers can enjoy this area with the aid of signposts that label some 55 different species of flowering shrubs and trees. Miles are also marked for those who wish to jog.

The trail outlines the Point Mallard peninsula and is bounded on one side by the Tennessee River and on two sides by Flint Creek. Beginning at the carpet golf course, the paved trail remains fairly level as it sweeps around the full golf course and ends at the 8th Street park entrance.

Trails in East Central Alabama

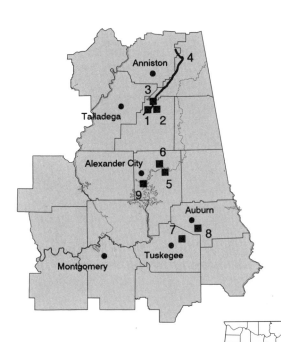

1. Lake Chinnabee Recreation Area
2. Cheaha Wilderness Area
3. Cheaha State Park
4. Pinhoti National Recreation Trail System
5. Horseshoe Bend National Military Park
6. Horseshoe Bend Trail
7. Bartram National Recreation Trail
8. Chewalla State Park
9. Wind Creek State Park

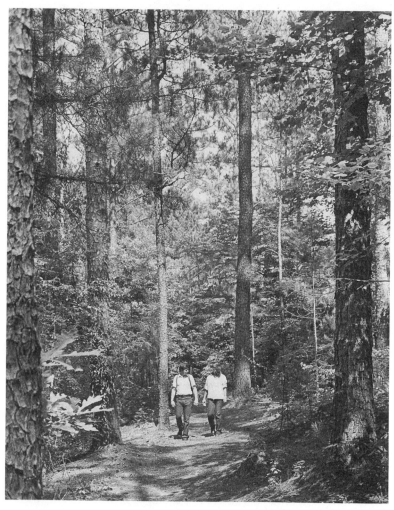

Pinhoti Trail, Talladega National Forest, Talladega Division (Photograph by Joy Patty, Courtesy the U.S. Department of Agriculture, Forest Service)

Lake Chinnabee Recreation Area

The Lake Chinnabee Recreation Area of the Talladega National Forest remains one of the prettiest of the U.S. Forest Service facilities in Alabama. Although one of the smallest campgrounds, it stays very busy because of its proximity to Cheaha State Park and the Pinhoti Trail System (see separate sections below). The Chinnabee area is named for an Indian who saved a group of settlers at Fort Lashley from a party of hostile Creek Indians. Sneaking through the band disguised in a hog skin, complete with legs, he returned with Andrew Jackson to defeat the Creeks. His grave lies 10 miles north of Talladega at McElderry Station.

The trail, which circles the lake, is open all year without charge. No physical aids exist but neither do any real hazards. The moderately easy trail is well traveled in most places but not extremely well marked.

The Lake Chinnabee Recreation Area can be found by traveling north from Talladega on U.S. 21 and taking County 42 (Cheaha Road) to the entrance signs.

Topos: Cheaha Mountain, Ironaton 1:24,000

Lake Chinnabee Trail

Length: 1.5 miles

Description: The trail starts across Cheaha Creek at the north end of the parking area and circles Lake Chinnabee. Hikers should not confuse this trail with the longer Chinnabee Silent Trail in the Cheaha Wilderness Area, which begins its ascent alongside the creek and departs from the south end of the parking area. Lake Chinnabee Trail mounts the hillside along the shoreline through tall pines and oak trees. Several small streams must be crossed, and wet-weather runoff ravines can be a problem for those not accustomed to rock hopping. Trillium and foxglove are just two of the wildflowers to look for in this area. The trail hugs the shoreline and loops through the campground at the south end of the lake to return to the service road and the parking area.

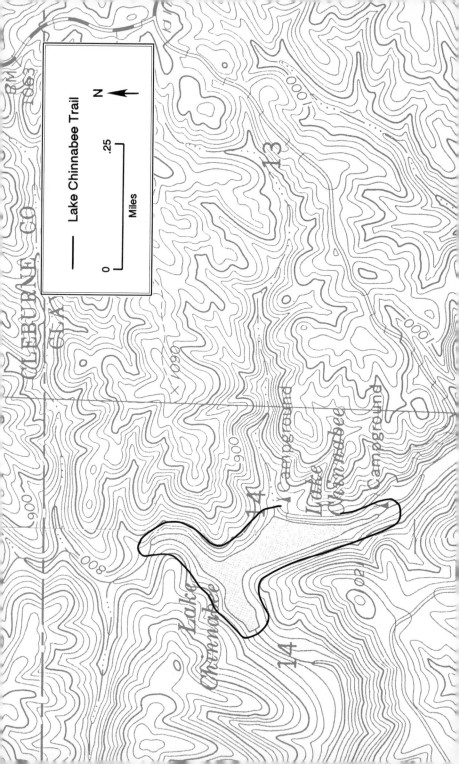

Cheaha Wilderness Area

The Cheaha Wilderness Area was established in 1983 to provide primitive outdoor experiences and solitude for visitors and to preserve natural ecological conditions in a portion of the Talladega National Forest. The 6,544-acre wilderness includes a part of the southernmost range of the Appalachian Mountains and contains over 1,000 acres above 2,000 feet in elevation.

Deer, opossum, fox, bobcat, weasel, turkey, and several species of hawks and owls all populate the forest. Because the area is easily accessible from nearby Cheaha State Park and its facilities, it rates as a popular destination for campers and hikers. Hiking in the wilderness area is rugged and rocky, making good shoes or hiking boots a necessity.

No fees are charged for hiking in the wilderness area; permits are necessary only during hunting season but are available at no charge from the district rangers. Forest service maps and additional information can be obtained from district ranger offices in Talladega, Heflin, or Montgomery.

Topos: Cheaha Mountain, Ironaton, Lineville West 1:24,000

Skyway Loop Trail

Length: 6 miles

Description: The trail's northern terminus forms at the southern parking lot of the Lake Chinnabee Recreation Area. The trail rises through the heavily wooded hillsides to a point overlooking the lake and then heads to the southwest in a very winding pathway, earning it a difficult rating because of its continuous undulations and its numerous stream crossings with no physical aids.

Approximately a mile after leaving the parking lot, the trail crosses FS 645. It soon intersects FS 645F and drops in elevation to ford Hubbard Creek, which usually flows year-round. Traveling near FS 633 for a mile, the path climbs again and follows the contours of the hillsides. At mile 4, Skyway Loop Trail descends into a small valley, where two wet-weather streams join to form Barbaree Creek. The trail follows the streambed for a mile before

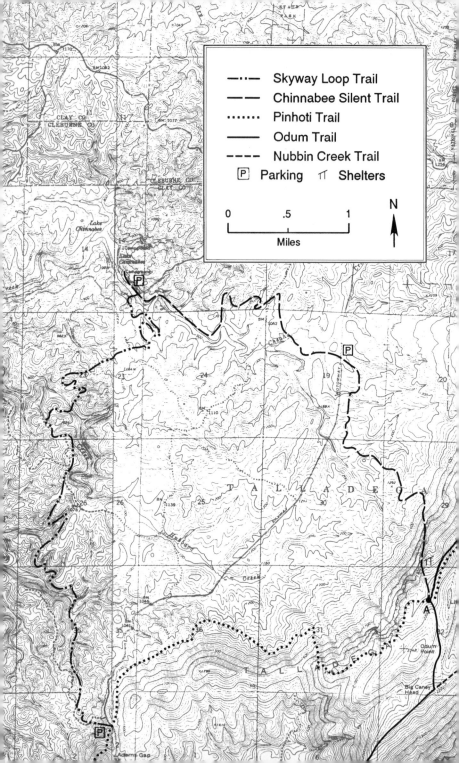

	Skyway Loop Trail
	Chinnabee Silent Trail
	Pinhoti Trail
	Odum Trail
	Nubbin Creek Trail
P	Parking π Shelters

0   .5   1
Miles

N

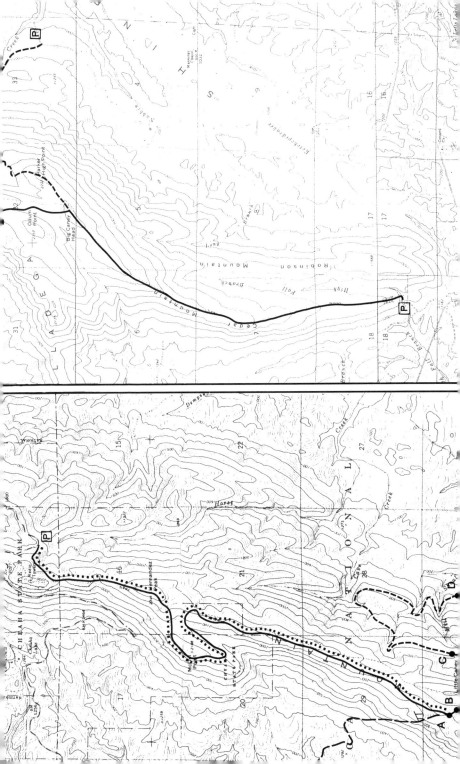

rising out of the depression to intersect with Pinhoti Trail near the Adams Gap parking area.

Skyway Loop Trail may be used in conjunction with Pinhoti and Chinnabee Silent trails to form a 17.5-mile loop suitable for a multiday trip.

Chinnabee Silent Trail

Length: 6 miles

Description: Chinnabee Silent Trail starts at the south parking area in the Chinnabee Recreation Area, another U.S. Forest Service facility. Named for the legendary Indian chief Chinnabee Selocta and built by Boy Scout Troop 29 of the Alabama Institute for the Deaf and Blind in Talladega, this trail may be the prettiest in the Talladega National Forest. The pathway earns its difficult rating on the steep and rugged stretch between the Skyway Motorway and its juncture with Pinhoti Trail (in the Pinhoti National Recreation Trail System) and Odum Trail. Small streams along the way may also present problems in wet weather, when crossings may be hazardous. Very few physical aids are provided.

After the trail leaves the parking area, it parallels Cheaha Creek, climbing gently and passing numerous swimming holes and small falls. As the pathway nears the halfway point at the Skyway Motorway (Forest Service [FS] 600), many hunters' footpaths appear, which may be confusing to those without a map and a compass. The trail crosses FS 600 near the Turnipseed hunting camp and bears west toward the ridgeline of Talladega Mountain. The last 1.5 miles of the trail creates a very steep and rocky climb, not for the faint of heart. The trail intersects Odum and Pinhoti trails near the Caney Head Shelter. From this point, the hiker can turn north and enter Cheaha State Park along Odum Trail (Pinhoti Trail also extends north along Odum Trail), turn south along the ridgeline of Cedar Mountain and end at High Falls near Pyriton, or travel southwest along Pinhoti Trail on Talladega Mountain toward Adams Gap.

Odum Trail

Length: 10.2 miles

Description: Odum Trail forms a part of the Pinhoti

Trail System, and for over 5 miles, the two coincide. As possibly the best-known trail in Alabama—having been literally the training ground for thousands of Boy and Girl Scouts and long-suffering Scout leaders—the trail's popularity stems largely from its location in Cheaha State Park, one of Alabama's most-visited state parks and the highest spot in Alabama.

Although overnight camping is not allowed inside the state park boundaries, many sites are available outside the park. Water is scarce along the trail, with the exception of a spring near Caney Head Shelter, and the water that is found should be treated to be potable. During dry weather, hikers are advised to carry a supply.

Odum Trail begins at the west end of the parking area near the park entrance off Alabama 49 Spur and climbs steeply up the side of Cheaha Mountain toward a set of radio towers—a moderately difficult hike because of the initial elevation gain in the first 1.5 miles. Rock scrambling is a necessity at several points as well, so hiking boots are strongly recommended. Offering some of the best views of the surrounding Talladega National Forest, the trail tops a rocky outcropping known as Hernandez Peak at the 1-mile point, which gives the hiker a chance to rest from the exertion and pull out the camera. Nearby McDill Point also makes a popular overlook, well worth lingering to see. The trail forms a 0.5-mile switchback and, a mile after passing the point, exits the state park and continues near the top of the ridge. The trail condition deteriorates along this stretch until one approaches Caney Head Shelter. Erosion and lack of trail maintenance have obliterated the trail surface for over a mile, so the faded tree markings are the hiker's only guide in some places. Caney Head Shelter, the halfway point on the trail, makes a popular overnight camping spot.

Shortly after leaving the shelter, Odum Trail intersects with Chinnabee Silent Trail where Pinhoti Trail diverges to the southwest. Two miles after the trails separate, the up-and-down nature of Odum Trail changes to a gentle descent from the ridgeline. At High Falls, steep metal steps beside the 30-foot cascade lead the hiker down into the small canyon formed long ago by High Falls Branch. The falls and large pool beneath a popular local swimming hole beckon hikers to take a cool rest stop or lunch break.

The trail exits through the canyon to an old forest service road and then to a parking area and camping site.

Nubbin Creek Trail

Length: 4.5 miles

Description: One of the newest in the Cheaha Wilderness, this constitutes the only trail to open up the east side of the wilderness area. As a newer trail, its surface is still good, and the pathway has not had a chance to become overgrown.

The trail, which begins at a parking area 5 miles north of Pyriton off Nubbin Creek Road, an offshoot of County 31, forms an easy to moderate trek, depending on the direction it is hiked. From the eastern parking area terminus to the western terminus at Odum Trail, it is more difficult because of the steepness of the grade that must be gained and its several stream crossings. The stream crossings still must be made from "top to bottom," but the downhill trek merely seems easier on the legs and lungs.

After leaving the parking area, the trail starts a gentle climb toward Mill Shoal Creek. Once paralleling the creek, it rises steeply, crossing the creek twice in the space of 0.25 mile and then turning sharply southwest. The path continues to ascend very steeply to Parker High Point, 2,232 feet in elevation, and 0.25 mile later intersects with Odum Trail.

Cheaha State Park

Cheaha State Park, one of the original 11 in Alabama, has been open continuously since 1933. Situated at the highest point in Alabama, at an elevation of 2,407 feet, the park was established by the Civilian Conservation Corps, as were so many others in the state park system. A museum dedicated to the Civilian Conservation Corps is located near the television towers atop the peak. The Cheaha Mountain Range forms the southernmost part of the Appalachian Mountain Range. The 2,719-acre park boasts complete facilities for both primitive and recreational vehicle camping on top of the mountain and by the lake, while a restaurant, motel, lodge, and housekeeping

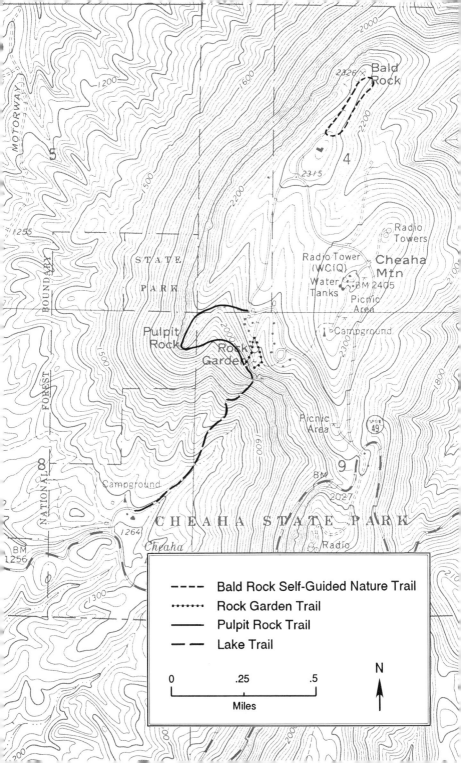

Bald Rock

2326

2000

1200

1600

2200

5

4

2315

Radio Towers

STATE

1255

Radio Tower (WCIQ)

Cheaha Mtn

PARK

Water Tanks

BM 2405

Picnic Area

Pulpit Rock

1500

Rock Garden

Campground

2200

1800

FOREST

1500

Picnic Area

SPUR 49

NATIONAL

1600

9

BM 2027

Campground

1264

CHEAHA STATE PARK

BM 1256

Cheaha

Radio

1300

2000

	Bald Rock Self-Guided Nature Trail
········	Rock Garden Trail
────	Pulpit Rock Trail
── ──	Lake Trail

N

0   .25   .5

Miles

cabins accommodate less adventurous groups. Day-use areas offer picnic shelters, playgrounds, and swimming and fishing at the lake. No fees are charged for day use and only small fees for camping.

The trails are all well marked and are easy to moderately strenuous. Since care should be taken in all rocky areas, good shoes or boots are recommended for short jaunts and are an absolute must for longer trips.

Located 25 miles north of Talladega and 17 miles west of Lineville, Cheaha State Park is open from dawn to dusk year-round. Scenic Alabama 49 makes a beautiful drive in the spring and even more so in the autumn, although the traffic can be bumper to bumper with sightseers.

Topo: Cheaha Mountain 1:24,000

Bald Rock Self-Guided Nature Trail

Length: 0.5 mile

Description: Bald Rock, the park's self-guided nature trail, takes about an hour to walk. This loop ranks as the easiest trail to walk in the park, so the whole family can make this excursion. On clear days, a visitor standing on top of Bald Rock may be able to see a radius of 75 miles. A brochure on the natural features is currently available, and signposts at each of the nature stations are in the process of being installed. The trail, beginning at the Bald Rock Lodge parking area, exemplifies the geology and the hardwoods and softwoods that predominate throughout the park. Spring, when the mountain laurel and wild hydrangea are in bloom, is an especially gorgeous time to visit.

Rock Garden Trail

Length: 0.25 mile

Description: This may well be the most scenic trail in a state park famous for its scenery. One can see miles of the Talladega National Forest, but the boulder-strewn mountainside with its wind-stunted pines is alone worth the price of admission. The trail runs short enough for almost any one to get in and out, although caution is advised in the scrambling that must be done over rocks and around boulders. The rock outcroppings at the end of the trail make popular rock-climbing areas and sunning spots in the spring and summers. At certain times of the year, a wet-weather spring cascades beside the trail, which can make the footing slippery. Rock Garden Trail begins off the service road to cabins 1 through 4 and enters and returns on the same route.

Pulpit Rock Trail

Length: 0.5 mile

Description: Pulpit Rock Trail, much like Bald Rock Trail in features, begins on the campground service road and provides an easy stroll through towering pines and mountain laurels. The last half of the trail winds around huge boulders to reach the brow of the mountain and the area known as Pulpit Rock. This is also considered a climber's playground, but those interested in less strenuous pursuits will enjoy the spectacular views from the rock outcroppings.

Lake Trail

Length: 1 mile

Description: Lake Trail branches off Rock Garden Trail at the top of the mountain and descends steeply to Cheaha Lake. For those familiar with the midwestern description of cold as a "three dog night," this trail may best be described as a "three mountain goat" trail. The first, very steep 0.5 mile meanders through huge rock formations and large stands of mountain laurel, while the next 0.25 mile parallels Cheaha Creek as it widens and becomes less steep. After the trail fords a small wet-weather stream, it levels out and creates an easy stroll to Lake Cheaha. To reverse direction and climb from Lake Cheaha to the top of the trail, the hiker can begin at the parking lot behind the bathhouse. One hiker who accompanied us suggested that anyone over the age of eight attempting the route from bottom to top should be advised to carry bottled oxygen.

EAST CENTRAL
ALABAMA

Pinhoti National
Recreation Trail System

In 1977, the Pinhoti Trail System was dedicated as the state's second National Recreation Trail (the Bartram near Tuskegee was the first) and has since become the state's most heavily traveled group of trails. The white turkey-foot blazes not only mark the pathway but also represent the Creek Indian name for this area, Pinhoti, literally "turkey home." One of Alabama's longest trail systems, it spans the Talladega District of the Talladega National Forest and furnishes some of the best and worst of Alabama hiking: the best of the hiking in the Pinhoti referring to the views from the mountaintops and a few areas still relatively untouched by the chainsaw forestry practices so prevalent over much of the state, and the worst being the clear-cut areas of the forest and the local practice of decorating every sign with a few bullet holes (thank goodness the light truck industry is not yet putting flame-thrower racks in pickups).

The trail system is rich in plant and animal life, with a portion of the trail located in the Choccolocco Wildlife Management Area. Lovers of wild food will find something to be gathered in every season, from morels and wintercress in the spring, to walnuts, persimmons, papaws, and muscadines in the fall. Deer, turkeys, opossums, bobcats, squirrels, and raccoons are common sights for those who are quiet and linger along the trail.

The only hazards in this area are the frequent stream crossings, which in wet weather can flood and become difficult, and the precipitous cliff overlooks, which require some care in footwork. Though generally available along the trail, water taken from nearby creeks and lakes should be filtered, treated chemically, or boiled to be safely drinkable.

Most of the trail is easily accessible via forest service (FS) roads, so one-way trips and loops of almost any length can be arranged. The trail descriptions are written from the perspective of north to south, which seems to be the route most often used. At this time, the Alabama Trails Association is working to develop the trail to the northeast, with the aim of eventually connecting it to the Appalachian Trail in northern Georgia. This newest por-

EAST CENTRAL
ALABAMA

88

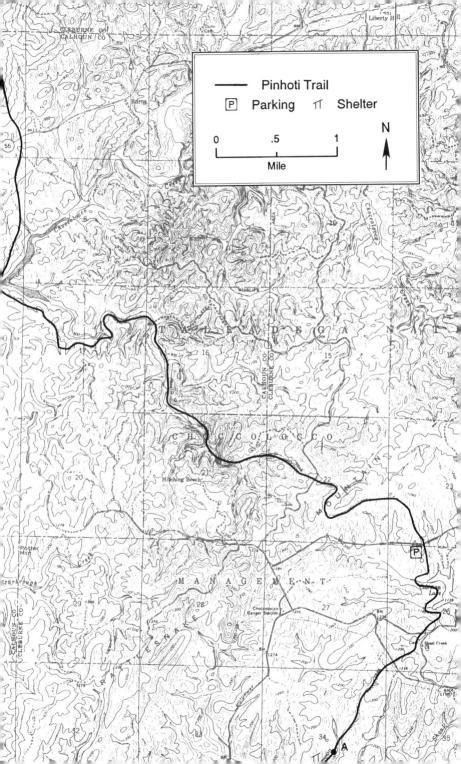

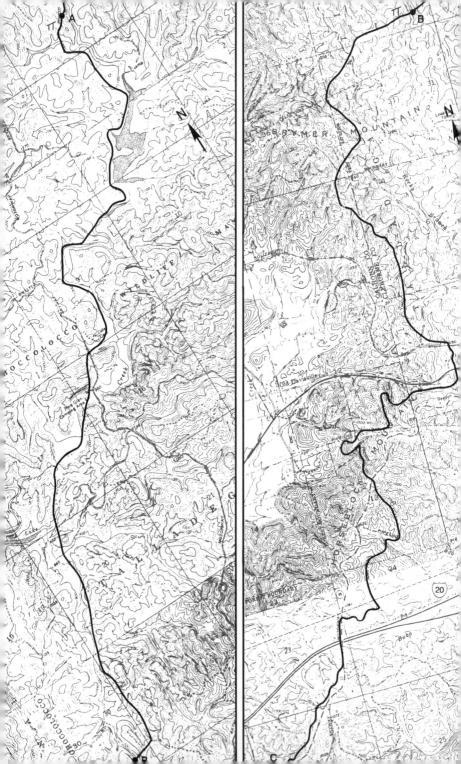

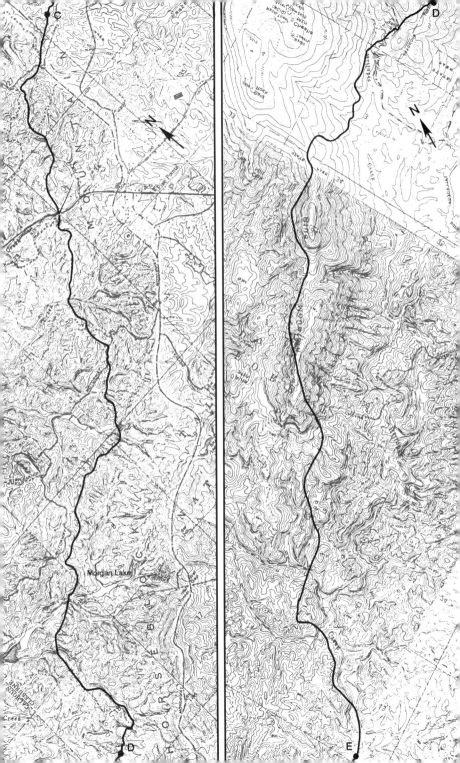

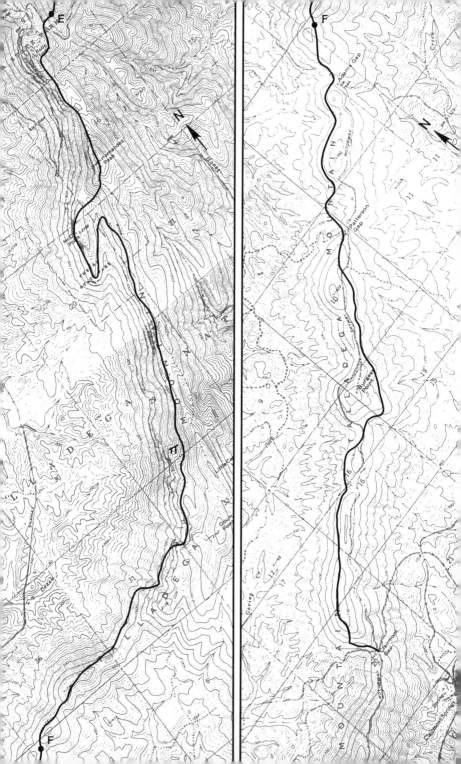

tion of the trail is currently under construction on private land east of the community of Piedmont in northern Calhoun County, just a few miles short of the Georgia border. This addition to the Pinhoti will take the trail across Oakey Mountain and will make a one-way trip from the Davis Mountain area along U.S. 278 to the southern terminus at Friendship, a total trail distance of 91 miles.

The trailhead for the proposed Davis Mountain/U.S. 278 section of the trail is located approximately 10 miles east of Piedmont near Davis Mountain. This area of the trail is not frequently used at this time, and there are no signs for the trailhead or parking areas for vehicles. Experienced hikers wishing to begin the Pinhoti Trail here should contact the Alabama Trails Association for exact information on trail conditions and parking for vehicles. At the time of this writing, the trail was passable, with some signs and turkey-foot markings. The area around Dugger Mountain was not a very pretty section of trail because of frequent deadfalls. Local forest service representatives were warning of some vehicle and sign vandalism near forest service road crossings. As the trail becomes used by more hikers, it is supposed that these incidents will decrease.

More information and forest service maps of the area are available for a small charge from the U.S. Forest Service supervisor's office in Montgomery or from the offices of the district ranger in Heflin or Talladega. No fees are charged for camping along the trail, but camping permits are required from the local ranger offices during hunting season (camping is permitted all along the trail except in Cheaha State Park). The Alabama Trails Association is also a valuable resource for up-to-date trail information. Those interested in information, joining the organization, or simply volunteering on the weekend trail maintenance or building crews should contact the association at P.O. Box 610311, Birmingham, Alabama 35261-0311 (205-836-9002).

County 55 to Coleman Lake

Length: 5.3 miles

Description: For the less adventurous or for those with larger groups and a larger number of vehicles, a better choice of route would be to start at County (CO) 55, where parking along the shoulder of the road is available, or at several nearby closed logging roads. Clear cutting has taken its toll in the Choccolocco Creek watershed, and this is not an easy entrance. Having entered the trail at the highway at the hiking sign 0.5 mile north of King Gap Road near Rabbittown, the hiker must climb a ridge through a bramble of briers and saplings, where most of the markings have been obliterated. The trail tops the ridge and drops to cross Choccolocco Creek near an old jeep trail, traveling southeast and paralleling a small run-off. Once the trail reaches the boundary into the Choccolocco Wildlife Management Area, it becomes much cleaner and its markings easier to follow. The trail crosses FS 540 and ends this section at FS 500 across from a parking area at the entrance to the Coleman Lake Recreation Area.

Topos: Jacksonville East, Piedmont Southeast 1:24,000

Coleman Lake to Lower Shoal Shelter

Length: 12 miles

Description: For many hikers, this will be the beginning of Pinhoti Trail until the Dugger Mountain section and northward are improved. The Coleman Lake Recreation Area, located off FS 500 near the Choccolocco game warden station, features boat ramps, recreational vehicle and primitive campgrounds, and fresh water and restroom facilities. The trail leaves the parking area on FS 500 and proceeds southward along the west end of the lake under a canopy of large pines, poplars, and dogwoods. Wide, rolling hillsides and a well-marked pathway, with few deadfalls at this writing, make for easy hiking throughout this section. With approximately 3.25 miles to Laurel Shelter, the trail crosses FS 553D and FS 553 and passes near Shoal Creek Church, one of only six hand-hewn log churches still standing in Alabama. Laurel Shelter nestles on a small creek in a low-lying area. The trail then runs along the shores of Sweetwater Lake, which has campsites and a boat-launching area but not much else in the way of facilities for campers. Following Shoal Creek for a mile or so until it passes Cole Cemetery, a final resting place for early settlers of the area, the Pinhoti intersects FS 500 and shortly thereafter enters Pine Glen Camping Area. Pine Glen offers drinking water, restrooms, campsites surrounded by sycamores and elms, and bass fishing for those with time to linger. After Pine Glen, the trail narrows, and since the area has been logged and burned in the not-so-distant past, the trees are sparser and the undergrowth heavier. More searching may be needed to find the turkey-track markings, especially where the trail crosses the frequent logging and jeep trails and signs have faded. Within 1.5 miles of traversing the wet bottomland near Highrock Lake, the pathway drops to a creek bank and passes Lower Shoal Shelter.

Topos: Jacksonville East, Piedmont Southeast, Choccolocco, Heflin 1:24,000

Lower Shoal Shelter to Interstate 20

Length: 12.2 miles

Description: After leaving Lower Shoal Shelter, the trail climbs the hill and crosses FS 531. Parts of this section too have been burned, which has given the undergrowth a chance to take over, but even though hiking is more difficult, the pathway is still obvious. Briers, blackberry vines, asters, foxgloves, and lobelia grow in abundance where the trail moves south toward U.S. 78. The trail crosses FS 523 and parallels FS 500 for 1.5 miles, until it intersects that road and then the railroad tracks at U.S. 78, which is also the northern terminus of Scenic Highway Alabama (AL) 49. The trail stays on the pavement across the highway and then exits the west side of AL 49 and reenters the woods. Because of the up-and-down nature of the terrain, this section ranks as one of the more difficult stretches of trail. Approximately a mile later, the trail crosses AL 49 once more and stays on the east side of the highway until it nears the AL 49 bridge over Interstate 20.

Topos: Choccolocco, Heflin, Oxford, Hollis Crossroads 1:24,000

Interstate 20 to Morgan Lake

Length: 9.5 miles

Description: This section of the trail parallels AL 49 for 2 miles before crossing FS 518 and then follows a small stream for a short distance before climbing over a ridge to intersect with U.S. 431 near mile marker 226. The trail jogs some 30 yards north up the highway before turning onto FS 585 and ascending back toward the woods. Instead of tracing the road around the first hairpin turn, the pathway exits to the southwest through the clearing. Since the trail is not well marked here, it may take some brush beating to find an indicator. After fording Little Hillabee Creek, the trail mounts the ridge and soon crosses FS 515. For the next 2 miles, the trail bounces up and down the ridgelines and wades through Hillabee Creek to intersect with CO 24 near Morgan Lake.

Several small stream crossings exist in this section (moderate rating) and in the next, so wet weather may be a consideration in choice of route. At high-water times of the year, hikers should be prepared to make alternate route choices.

Topos: Oxford, Hollis Crossroads 1:24,000

Morgan Lake to Cheaha State Park

Length: 12.2 miles

Description: In the past 5 years, this section of the Pinhoti has suffered through two tornados and a forest fire; thus conditions on this stretch of trail are rough, to say the least. At the time of this writing, the forest service is considering rerouting and remarking the trail, so hikers should check with local rangers for latest information.

The trail intersects CO 24 and enters another segment of rugged up-and-down Smoky Mountain–like terrain (moderately difficult) as it wanders over Horseblock Mountain. Since the trail is much narrower here in the Hillabee Creek watershed, usage is much lighter. Pine trees still predominate, but occasional stands of oak and sassafras add color to the forest. Approximately halfway through this portion, the trail dips into a 10-foot-wide dirt rut, euphemistically referred to as Cheaha Road, and rises steeply up the side of Blue Mountain. The path clings to the top of the mountain for over a mile before dropping slightly to enter Cheaha State Park. The Pinhoti continues to hover around a 2,000-foot elevation on this side of Cheaha Mountain, Alabama's highest peak at 2,405 feet.

Topos: Oxford, Hollis Crossroads, Cheaha Mountain 1:24,000

Cheaha State Park to Adams Gap

Length: 10.9 miles

Description: This moderate section of trail intersects AL 49 Spur near the parking area for Odum Scout Trail. The Pinhoti joins Odum Scout Trail for the next 5.4 miles, rising steeply up the side of Cheaha Mountain and proceeding south along the ridgeline. The trail soon crosses the rock outcropping known as Hernandez Peak and for the next mile provides the best views of these rugged mountains along Pinhoti Trail. Shortly after passing McDill Point, another lookout with a panoramic view, the pathway leaves the boundaries of Cheaha State Park and continues its way along Talladega Mountain. This section of the trail is higher in elevation and relatively dry, so hikers should be prepared to carry water. Caney Head Shelter, the halfway point of this section of the trail, does have a spring nearby, but during dry weather, it can disappear.

Shortly after passing the shelter, the Pinhoti intersects Chinnabee Silent Trail, which turns right toward Chinnabee Lake some 6 miles west, and Odum Scout Trail, which climbs the ridge to the left. The Pinhoti goes straight and traces the ridgeline to drop gently toward Adams Gap, where the trail cuts across the unpaved and semipassable Skyway Motorway (FS 600).

Topos: Cheaha Mountain, Ironaton, Clairmont Springs 1:24,000

Adams Gap to Clairmont Gap

Length: 6 miles

Description: Having traversed FS 600, the trail clings to the side of the ridges along the west side of Talladega Mountain until Patterson Gap, after which it continues to drop intermittently, signaling the beginning of the gentle hills of central Alabama. The forest becomes

EAST CENTRAL ALABAMA

97

more open, since this area has been logged heavily in the past and pines now predominate. Fruit lovers will find muscadine vines, huckleberries, blueberries, blackberries, gooseberries, wild strawberries, and even persimmons near the pathway in these dry upland woods. The trail zigzags beside the Skyway Motorway (FS 600) for the next 3 miles, until it concludes at the Friendship Church at Clairmont Gap, 1 mile north of Clairmont Springs. This final section of the Pinhoti Trail ranks as a moderately easy hike.

A pleasant continuation of the trip is to follow the Skyway Motorway down Talladega Mountain from Clairmont Gap to the Talladega Creek Bridge at the base of the mountain. Trail building continues to extend the Pinhoti to Chandler Springs, but since erosion has presented a problem for these efforts, the road is a better alternative. These additional 4.7 miles are worth the extra time and energy.

Topos: Ironaton, Clairmont Springs 1:24,000

Horseshoe Bend National Military Park

The Battle of Horseshoe Bend in March of 1814 cost the Creek Nation over 1,000 lives and eventually led to their ceding to the United States some 20 million acres of land, part of which later became the state of Alabama. For Andrew Jackson, who led the Tennessee militia in the battle, the decisive victory was the first step on his road to the White House.

The park today offers a visitor's center containing exhibits and slide programs on Creek Indian culture, pioneer life, and the Creek War of 1813–14. Special tours for groups can be arranged with the superintendent of the park. An interpretive drive loops for 3 miles through the park, with markers to help the visitor envision the battle, and the nature trail allows the foot traveler a chance to stroll across the battlefield among the gun placements. A picnic area, restrooms, and drinking water complete the park's facilities. Horseshoe Bend National Military Park, located 12 miles north of Dadeville on Alabama 49, is open from 9 A.M. to 6 P.M. daily. While this park has no camping area, facilities are available at nearby Wind Creek

EAST CENTRAL
ALABAMA

98

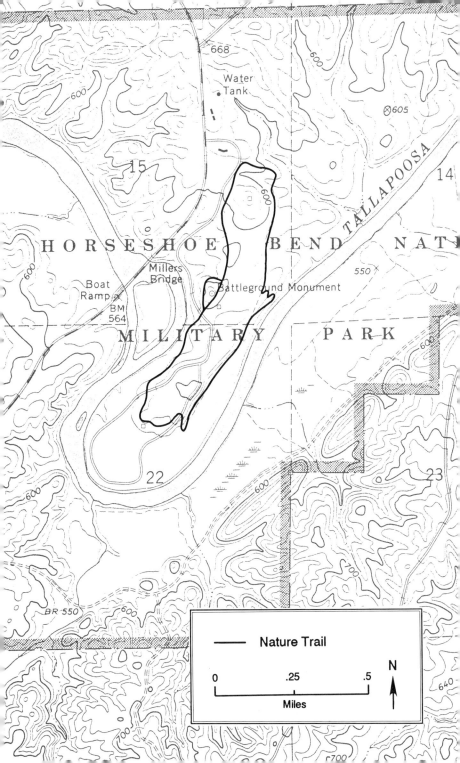

State Park, 6 miles south of Alexander City. For more information, contact the superintendent, Horseshoe Bend National Military Park, Route 1, Box 103, Daviston, Alabama 36256.

Topo: Buttston 1:24,000

Nature Trail

Length: 2.8 miles

Description: The Nature Trail, an easy, relatively flat pathway with interpretive signs and shelters, describes the events of the Battle of Horseshoe Bend. At the parking area near driving tour stop 1, the trail enters the woods to begin the first part of the loop past a small cannon at the top of Gun Hill. It then drops off the high ground to skirt the edge of the battlefield for a mile and travel into the curve of the horseshoe itself where the encampment of Tohopeka, an Indian refugee village, existed in 1814. Turning north, the trail moves to the edge of the Tallapoosa River for 0.25 mile before returning to complete the loop at Cotton Patch Hill, where Jackson's troops awaited deployment on the morning of the battle.

Horseshoe Bend Trail

This Tallapoosa County trail wanders through wooded hillsides and across small streams, tracing the path chosen by Andrew Jackson and his Tennessee volunteers on their way to the Battle of Horseshoe Bend with the Creek Indians. The trail ends at the visitor's center at Horseshoe Bend National Military Park, which commemorates the site where General Jackson defeated the Creek Indian Confederacy and opened the Southwest for settlement by the pioneers.

Horseshoe Bend Trail, currently administered and maintained by the Tukabatchee Council Boy Scouts of America, is not in good shape. Trash and woodcutting have made sections of the trail a less than peak outdoors experience, encouraging a certain nostalgia for the period of the Indians. One primitive campsite exists on the trail, but for other facilities, the hiker must retreat to the military park, Wind Creek State Park, Dadeville, or Alexander City. Water is available from several small streams and

EAST CENTRAL ALABAMA

100

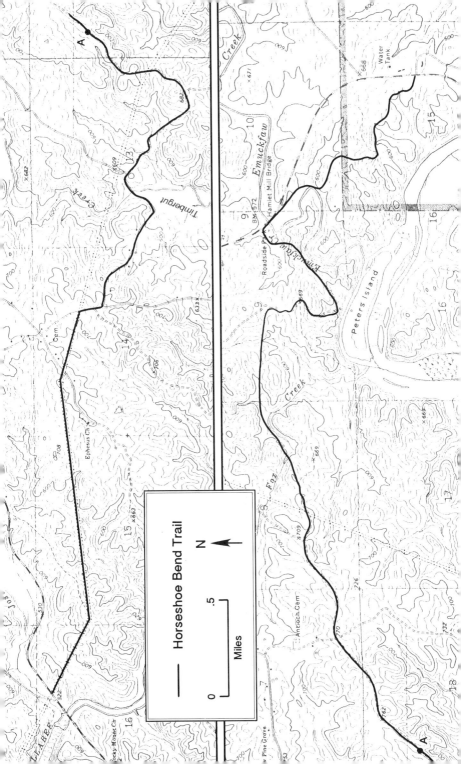

Horseshoe Bend Trail

N

Miles

0   .5

from a rudimentary pump at the overnight campsite, but these are not safe sources; all water must be boiled, filtered, or chemically treated before drinking or must be carried in by the hiker. For more information, contact the Boy Scout Tukabatchee Council, Carter Hill Road, Montgomery, Alabama.

Topo: Jackson's Gap 1:24,000

Horseshoe Bend Trail

Length: 10 miles

Description: The trailhead is located slightly east of Hillabee Creek on Alabama (AL) 22, 5 miles northeast of Alexander City. Cars may be left roadside at AL 22, at the owner's risk, or at the national park visitor's center, which is locked overnight. The trail follows the clear-cut area along the Alabama Power Company electrical lines for 2 miles. After intersecting with the second paved road, the trail veers away from the power lines and turns south along the road for a short distance and then back to the east (left) for 0.5 mile. The paved road ends at the crossing of Timbergut Creek, and the trail turns to clay for several miles. Well marked with orange blazes throughout most of this area, the trail is a moderate hike, with much of it along old jeep tracks or pulpwood truck roads.

After the bridge over Timbergut Creek, the road mounts a hill and turns right. At approximately mile 6 on the trail, 0.5 mile later, the pathway turns left, still following the road, and soon passes under the power lines again and climbs the hill. A mile or so later, it crosses a clay road and continues east under another set of power lines toward the overnight campsite.

Passing the campsite, the trail jogs downhill, crossing the low-lying area surrounding Fox Creek. This creek bottom is notorious for snakes, so hikers must exercise caution, especially around underbrush. The trail rejoins a jeep track that leads south toward the Tallapoosa River for 0.25 mile, turns back to the east just before the riverbanks, and then enters the forest. Near Emuckfaw Creek, Horseshoe Bend Trail intersects with AL 49 at a roadside park on the creek. Blazes lead hikers through another unofficial overnight camp, along jeep trails, and on to Horseshoe Bend National Military Park.

Bartram National Recreation Trail

This Macon County national forest area is rich not only in scenery but in history as well. Over 200 years ago, William Bartram became America's first native-born artist-naturalist. He traveled extensively throughout the Southeast, and his journals were later published as *Bartram's Travels,* the classic volume that provides, in some cases, the only insight into the environment of this area during the 18th century. Bartram spent Christmas Eve of 1775 in what later became the Tuskegee National Forest, and on the bicentennial of that date, the secretary of agriculture declared a portion of the same area as a national recreation trail. However, the Quaker naturalist was not the only traveler along these trails. The passageways through this forest area had long been used by the Talisi Indians, Spanish explorers from Mexico, and eventually the English in trading and peace negotiations with the Indians.

Tuskegee National Forest is located near Interstate 85 (I-85) between Montgomery and Auburn. The terrain of this easy trail is rolling and not especially steep, but some care must be taken in crossing streams and jumping over wet spots. Bartram Trail has several access points with nearby parking areas, but those wishing to hike the entire trail will find it easier to start at the upper northeastern end and proceed to the west. The Tsinia Wildlife Viewing Area, located about a mile from the western end of the trail, is well worth the visitor's time and effort. Quiet observers, in the spring and autumn especially, will see a variety of waterfowl moving through the area and a host of local creatures, such as deer, squirrels, and turkeys, going about their daily business. In this area, hunting, fishing, trapping, and pets are not allowed.

The Taska Recreation Area also lies in the vicinity and serves as a day-use area with picnic tables, grills, and a replica of Booker T. Washington's birthplace nearby. No fees are charged for usage of any of the national forest facilities, and the area is open to hikers year-round. Overnight camping is allowed along the trail, but heavy usage and the shortness of the trail generally discourage this practice. Mountain bikers too find the trail appealing, so this traffic is heavy as well, and additional care should be

EAST CENTRAL ALABAMA

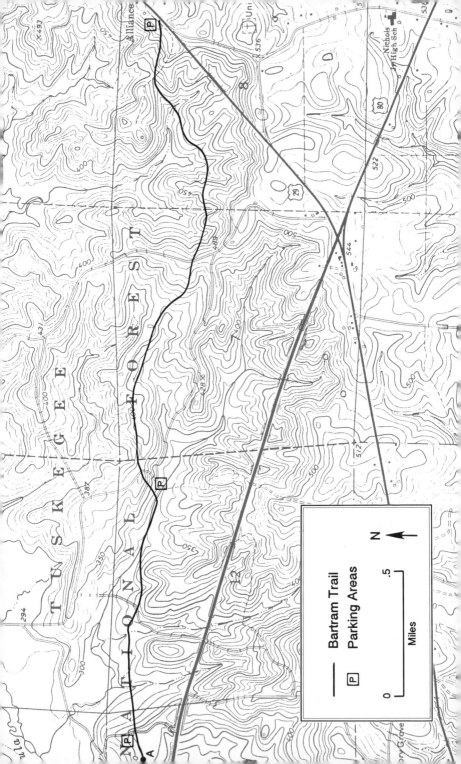

Bartram Trail
Parking Areas

N

.5

Miles

0

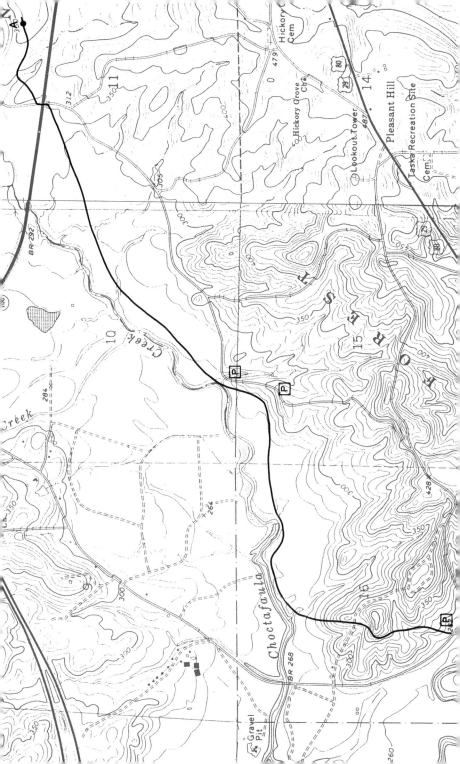

taken to avoid collisions. Bartram Trail is located off U.S. 29 east of exit 42 on I-85.

Topos: Tuskegee, Little Texas 1:24,000

Bartram Trail

Length: 8.5 miles

Description: The trail begins in the parking area off U.S. 29 in the eastern end of the Tuskegee National Forest and travels through rolling hillsides and tall trees for 2.3 miles to Forest Service (FS) Road 906. After traversing the road, the trail ascends a hill and fords a small stream with a footbridge. Throughout this area, dogwoods, hickories, poplars, and sassafras trees form a canopy for the trail, and wildflowers, including coneflowers and mistflowers, dot the sunnier spots. The trail then crosses FS 905 and, after another mile or so, enters a parking area near a ranger office.

The trail soon intersects Alabama 186 and starts again on the other side of the highway. The terrain changes to bottomland as the path nears Choctafaula Creek and passes two parking areas along FS 900. A mile after passing the parking areas, a short side trail leads to the creek and its beach, which seem to call the hiker for a quick rest and a chance to soak hot feet. Oak and pine trees abound in the heavily forested bottom where the pathway parallels the creek. The trail climbs the hills for the last mile or so to end at the parking area at FS 913.

Chewacla State Park

Built in the 1930s under the Civilian Conservation Corps program, Chewacla State Park is one of the original Alabama state parks. The 696-acre park, located 3 miles south of Auburn off U.S. 29 with access from Interstate 85 and open daily all year, has vacation cottages, tent and trailer campsites, canoe and paddleboat rentals, and fishing and swimming facilities. Chewacla, a Creek Indian word meaning "raccoon town," abounds with wildlife, especially deer. Since the park lies within bicycling distance of the Auburn University campus, it rates as a popular spot with students.

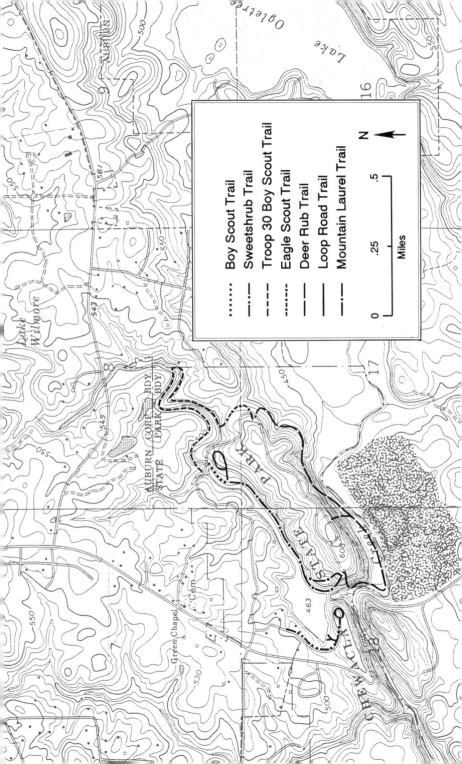

Boy Scout Trail
Sweetshrub Trail
Troop 30 Boy Scout Trail
Eagle Scout Trail
Deer Rub Trail
Loop Road Trail
Mountain Laurel Trail

N

0   .25   .5

Miles

Lake Ogletree

16

Lake
Wilmore

17

AUBURN GORE BDY
STATE PARK BDY

STATE PARK

Green Chapel

Cem

18

CHEWACLA

None of the hikes through Chewacla State Park are long, but some can be steep and, in places, poorly marked. All the paths interconnect, except Sweetshrub Trail, so it is possible to make a longer day by combining, for example, Deer Rub Trail with Mountain Laurel Trail. Information sheets and maps are available at park headquarters, which levies a small fee for day use.

Topo: Auburn 1:24,000

Boy Scout Trail

Length: 0.4 mile

Description: This easy, well-marked trail starts on the west side of the stone bridge along the entrance road and runs into Sweetshrub Trail.

Sweetshrub Trail

Length: 0.3 mile

Description: The park's interpretive nature trail, Sweetshrub makes an easy loop that starts and ends at the Lower Shelter. Information sheets highlighting the plants and trees along this path are available at park headquarters. Some guideposts with signs are also present, but many had fallen into disrepair at the time of our visit.

Troop 30 Boy Scout Trail

Length: 2 miles

Description: Slightly more difficult to hike than Sweetshrub Trail or Boy Scout Trail, this path represents one of the prettiest in the park. It begins on the north side of the stone bridge on Murphy Drive, follows Moore's Mill Creek to the boundary of the park, and then stops. As an alternative, the hiker can cross one of the stone dams and follow the trail back to the bridge. Owing to the nearness of the stream, the path is generally damp, so footing can be hazardous.

Eagle Scout Trail

Length: 0.7 mile

Description: Easy, relatively well marked Eagle Scout Trail branches off Troop 30 Boy Scout Trail on the east side of Moore's Mill Creek and ends on the logging road across from the Walnut Shelter. It can also be reached from the parking lot located between the Walnut and Creek shelters.

Deer Rub Trail

Length: 2 miles

Description: The trail starts at the Upper Pavilion, descends steeply to Chewacla Creek, and parallels the creek to the logging road across from Walnut Shelter. Although the path is marked, the steepness of the terrain and a few badly eroded spots make it more difficult to hike. It is also possible to enter the trail from the east side of the overlook on the Upper Pavilion circle. This entry too is steep, and erosion has taken its toll.

Loop Road Trail

Length: 0.3 mile

Description: This trail, a paved maintenance road that has been closed to motor traffic, takes a pleasurable stroll to the picturesque Chewacla Dam Falls.

Mountain Laurel Trail

Length: 1.3 miles

Description: The moderately easy Mountain Laurel Trail, with several well-marked entrances at the Upper Pavilion area, travels steeply down to Chewacla Falls, a popular sunning spot in spring, and then curves around the shoreline of Chewacla Lake to reach the stone bridge on Murphy Drive. Several connecting trails also loop this path back to the Upper Pavilion for a longer and more strenuous hike. Even though the connections are not marked, the various pathways are well traveled and thus easily distinguished.

Wind Creek State Park

Rambling along the shores of Lake Martin, this state park is geared primarily to water and boating activities. But in addition to its fishing piers, marina, boat ramps, and

EAST CENTRAL ALABAMA

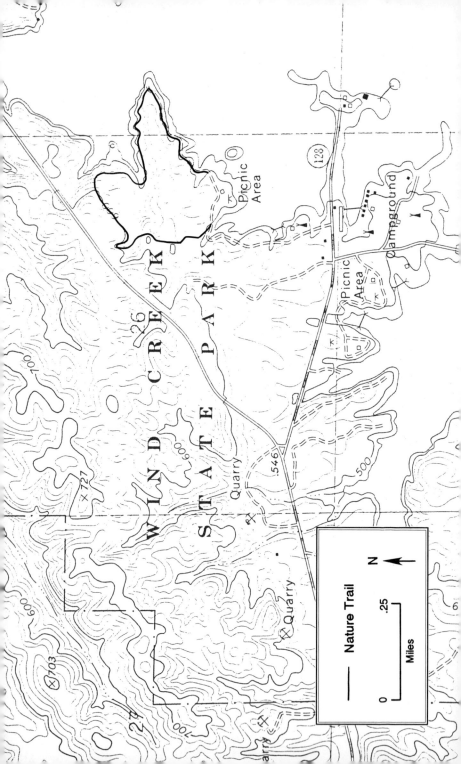

beaches, Wind Creek State Park does boast a short easy nature trail. Camping, both recreational vehicle and primitive, is available for a fee, as are boat rentals and boat storage at the marina. Summer always finds overflow crowds of campers and day-use visitors eager to escape the heat in Alabama or to hold family reunions at one of the many picnic pavilions available by reservation. Even with overflow crowds, this is one of the cleaner and better-kept parks in the system.

Autumn and spring, when the temperatures are cooler, figure as the best times for walking in the park, and small mammals and deer are almost always seen. The relatively clear nature trail is well marked with yellow blazes. Lush shallow ravines with mushrooms and ferns line the trail, and wild ginger and muscadine vines pepper the hillsides.

Wind Creek State Park, situated off Alabama 63 and County 128, 7 miles southeast of Alexander City, is open daily from 7 A.M. to 9 P.M. with a small entrance fee.

Topo: Our Town 1:24,000

Nature Trail

Length: 2 miles

Description: The trail begins at the end of the service road near the North Picnic Area, where parking is available. The trail slowly mounts along the edge of the lake on a wide level pathway for 0.5 mile before turning northward. Still very evident through the tall pine and oak trees, the pathway rises more steeply and veers away from the lake.

At the 1-mile mark, the trail turns southwest for a short distance, intersects an old jeep trail, and drops along several small ravines to end finally at the service road. The hiker must walk 100 yards northeast along the road to complete the loop.

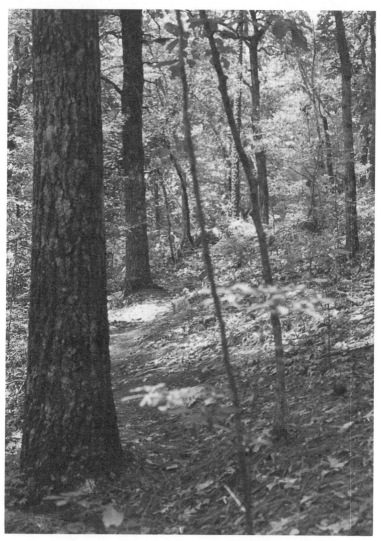

Payne Lake Recreation Area, Talledega National Forest, Oakmulgee Division (Photograph by Mike Sharpe)

Trails in West Central Alabama

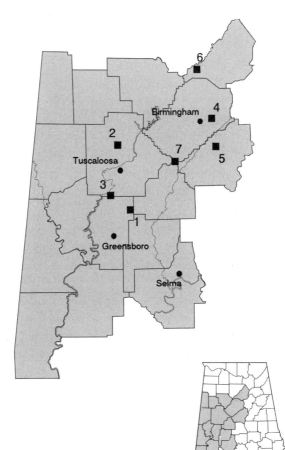

1. Payne Lake Recreation Area
2. Lake Lurleen State Park
3. Moundville Archaeological Park
4. Ruffner Mountain Nature Center
5. Oak Mountain State Park
6. Rickwood Caverns State Park
7. Tannehill Historical State Park

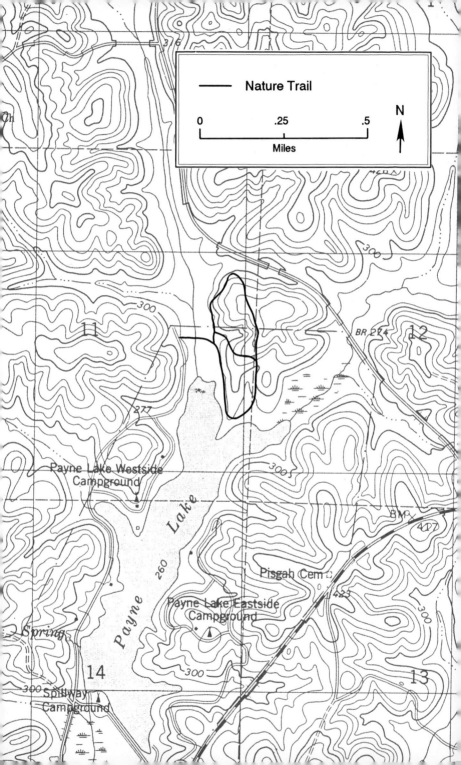

Payne Lake Recreation Area

Payne Lake Recreation Area, the only public-use area in the Oakmulgee Ranger District of the Talladega National Forest, attracts visitors more interested in fishing than in camping, but a small trail system does exist for those wishing to get a closer look at the plants and animals of west Alabama. Established in 1965 in a cooperative effort by the forest service and the Garden Club of Alabama, the trail is easily walked and offers handrails and wooden walkways where necessary in the low-lying areas. A few of the original nature identification signs still exist, but most have been defaced or removed, apparently in a cooperative effort by the irresponsible.

Payne Lake Recreation Area, located 15 miles north of Greensboro on Forest Service 714 off Alabama 25, sports recreational vehicle and primitive camping sites, a boat ramp, fishing and swimming areas, drinking water, restrooms, and picnic tables. Day-use and camping fees are charged, but no fee is levied for the nature trail.

Topo: Payne Lake 1:24,000

Nature Trail

Length: 1 mile

Description: This loop actually comprises an interconnected set of four small paths that begin at the parking area beyond the Payne Lake Westside Campground. A signboard at the trailhead discloses the layout of the paths and their distances. After following the boardwalk a short distance, the trail branches to the left north and to the right south. Following the south trail takes the hiker toward the lake and into the low-lying woods near the creek. Solomon seal, wild oats, partridge berry, wild ginger, and cypress trees flourish along the trail. The pathway soon turns and rises out of the lake basin to skirt the top of the ridge along the remnants of an old logging railroad bed. The higher ground is home to tall poplars, bays, beeches, oaks, and several species of pine. The trail then tops the ridge and drops toward the other small creek that brackets this trail. Onward 0.25 mile, the loop is completed, and the pathway back to the signboard is marked.

WEST CENTRAL ALABAMA

Lake Lurleen State Park

Besides hosting a series of hiking trails, Lake Lurleen State Park provides a variety of other recreational activities. The 250-acre lake is stocked with game fish, and both recreational vehicle and primitive campsites are available. A beach area and a large day-use area are maintained, and canoes and fishing boats can be rented.

The trails surrounding Lake Lurleen, named for the late Governor Lurleen B. Wallace, feature a large number of hardwoods, as well as several varieties of pines and maples. In the spring, purple anise and wild azaleas dot the hillsides, and low-lying areas boast several species of fern. Even though self-guiding, the hiking trails are not well marked and, in some seasons of the year, are not well traveled, so some care should be exercised. The area is hilly, and good shoes will be helpful.

The park, open daily from 7 A.M. to 9 P.M. with a small usage fee, lies within the Coker community, 15 miles northwest of Tuscaloosa on U.S. 82 off County 21. Park area maps are available at the entrance or at the camp store and the manager's office.

Topo: Lake Lurleen 1:24,000

Red Trail

Length: 0.8 mile

Description: Beginning behind the outdoor chapel on Lake Lurleen Drive across from the playground, the trail continues in a moderately steep climb over several small hills to one of the highest points in the park. The abundance of red maples and wildflowers makes the Red Trail–White Trail loop an easy and colorful walk. This trail also intersects Yellow Trail.

Freddie B. Smith Trail

Length: 1.2 miles

Description: The longest individual trail in the park, Smith Trail originates at the lakeshore just below the entrance to the park and hugs the shoreline for its entire length. It represents one of the more pleasant trails for most of the year, but when the small flies that the bass love

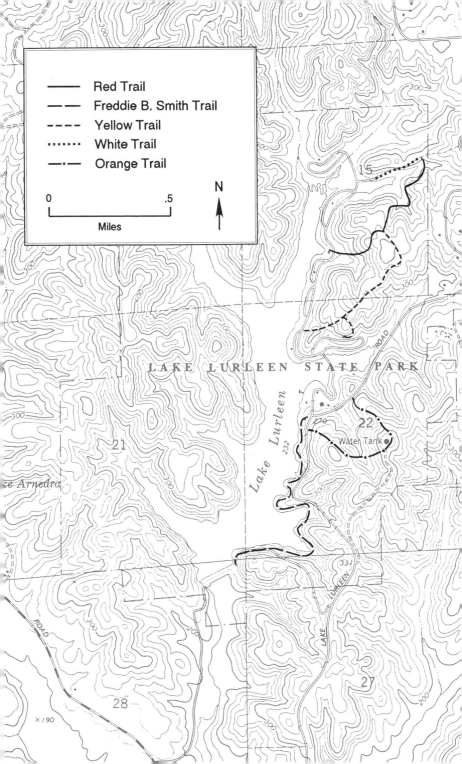

Red Trail
Freddie B. Smith Trail
Yellow Trail
White Trail
Orange Trail

0 .5

Miles

N

LAKE LURLEEN STATE PARK

Lake Lurleen

Water Tank

15

22

21

ce Arnedra

300

270

232

331

28

27

× / 90

ROAD

ROAD

LAKE

LURLEEN

are swarming, it is best to avoid this particular stroll. This trail ends at the dam, where hikers can retrace their steps or return on the dirt road that leads back to Lake Lurleen Road.

Yellow Trail

Length: 0.7 mile
Description: Starting across the road from the beach swimming area, this trail either forms a brief 0.3-mile jaunt to end at the campsite 1–29 area, or it climbs steeply up the ridge to join Red Trail. Portions of the Yellow, Red, and White trails may be linked to form a 1.25-mile hike, which begins where Yellow Trail originates, continues on Red Trail, and joins White Trail to end at the parking area where White Trail starts.

White Trail

Length: 0.3 mile
Description: The shortest of the nature trails starts at the end of the parking area between campsite areas 41–59 and 60–86. The trailhead is well marked, and the pathway itself traces an old timber track, so it is wide and easy to travel. It ascends gently through hardwoods to the boundary of the park, where the track is cabled off. One can return to the parking area at this point or join Red Trail for a return to the park service road.

Orange Trail

Length: 0.6 mile
Description: Orange Trail begins and ends along Lake Lurleen Road outside the entrance to the park itself. It starts just before the turnoff to the park and rises along an old access road to circle the water tower and return to the road after the turnoff. Although a fairly easy climb, it is not well marked after the entrance and is overgrown with brush in some spots.

Moundville Archaeological Park

WEST CENTRAL ALABAMA

One of the most interesting prehistoric areas in Alabama, Moundville Archaeological Park was once the

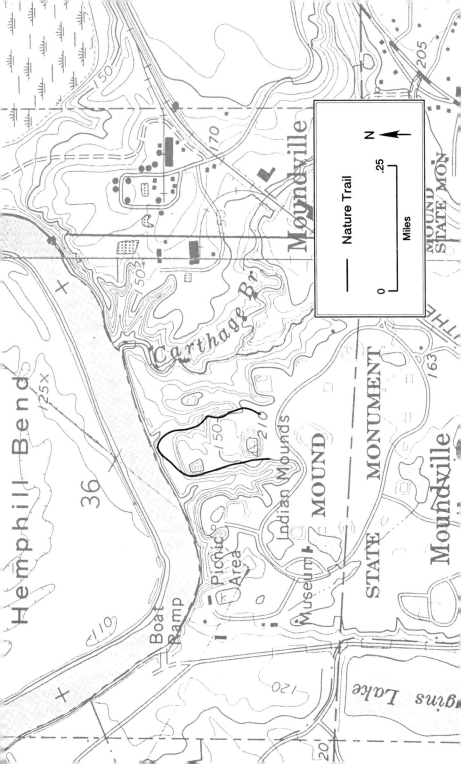

location of a large settlement of southeastern Indians between A.D. 1000 and 1500. This area on the banks of the Black Warrior River has also received national acclaim as the site of one of the largest Indian mounds in the United States, a 60-foot-high earthenwork, along with some 20 other mounds. The museum in the park houses collections of artifacts of several hundred archaeological sites excavated since 1929 by The University of Alabama and features reconstructions of these excavated sites. Facsimiles of prehistoric buildings nearby and life-size Indian replicas portray daily activities and ceremonies.

The park is located 13 miles south of Tuscaloosa off Alabama 69, 1 mile west of Moundville. Camping areas, both recreational vehicle and primitive, are available, as are picnic facilities and wheelchair access. The museum and camping areas charge a small fee. The museum is open 9 A.M. to 5 P.M. seven days a week except major winter holidays, and the park is open from 5 A.M. to 9 P.M. on the same schedule. For more information, contact Moundville Archaeological Park, P.O. Box 66, Moundville, Alabama 35474.

Topo: Fosters 1:24,000

Nature Trail

Length: 1 mile

Description: This easy, self-guiding trail begins at the largest mound and temple reconstruction area, meanders through a wooded area yet to be fully explored by archaeologists, and ends at an overlook on the banks of the Black Warrior River. Work is currently under way to lengthen the trail into a loop that returns to the mound area.

Ruffner Mountain Nature Center

The Ruffner Mountain Nature Center effort was initiated in 1977 with the acquisition of an abandoned house and 28 acres of overgrown hillside. The center today encompasses approximately 500 acres and over 1,200 members interested in retaining open spaces and a sense of nature even in the heart of urban clutter. The three

WEST CENTRAL
ALABAMA

120

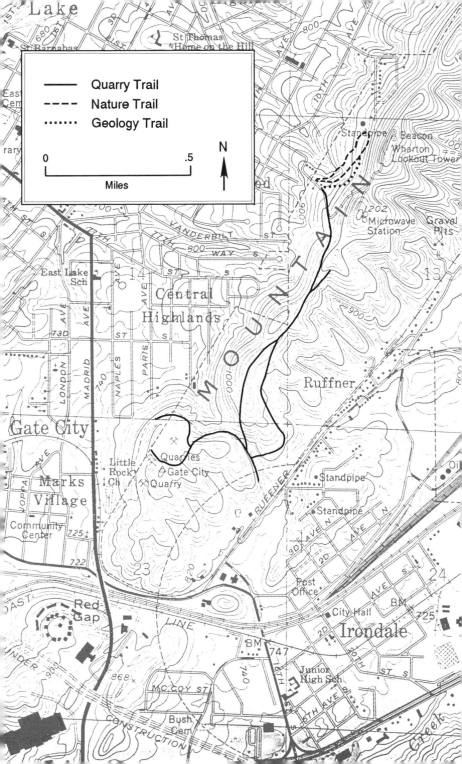

longer trails exhibit the wildlife and the geology of the area and showcase the large variety of trees and plants indigenous to the Birmingham area. A very short path, called the Wildflower Garden Trail, also winds behind the nature center.

The center, open until 8 P.M. from May to October and until 5 P.M. from November to April, charges no entrance fee and only a small fee for the nature guides. The center can be reached by taking Oporto Road from Interstate 20 and then going north to Rugby Avenue and 81st Street. From Interstate 59, the 77th Street exit can be taken and Rugby Avenue reached from that side.

Those interested in further information should contact Ruffner Mountain Nature Center, 1214 South 81st Street, Birmingham, Alabama 35306.

Topo: Irondale 1:24,000

Quarry Trail

Length: 3 miles

Description: This loop, the most interesting and varied of the trails here on Ruffner Mountain, does some backtracking on itself. The trail begins beyond the gate off the service road behind the nature center. While relatively level, the trail does have some steep sections, which the view of Birmingham makes worthwhile. The same trees that characterize the area around the nature center grow here too. Poplars, hackberries, black cherries, dogwoods, pines, persimmons, hickories, oaks, and sassafras trees are all identified for the hiker with the aid of trail markers and a guidebook obtained from the center. The abandoned late 1800s limestone quarry squats roughly a mile from the center, and the hiker can traverse the bottom of the quarry looking for fossils in the rock. After enjoying the view of Birmingham, the visitor returns to the start roughly along the same pathway. Benches along the way provide spots for resting or spying on the many creatures that inhabit this area.

Nature Trail

Length: 1 mile

Description: This easy, short trail winds through the old hardwood forest of Ruffner Mountain. The trail begins at the edge of the parking area just below the center, climbs slightly up the ridge, and then loops back to the center. Most of the trees are oak and hickory, with a sprinkling of pines, dogwoods, hawthorns, and persimmons. The walking is easy, although care should be taken around the sandstone and limestone outcroppings, especially during wet periods. Numbered stations correspond with the nature guide which can be obtained from the center.

Geology Trail

Length: 0.5 mile
Description: The Geology Trail highlights the natural geological processes that go virtually unnoticed from generation to generation. This trail starts near the Wildflower Garden Trail at the rear of the nature center and ascends slightly up the ridge to intersect the Nature Trail. The force of erosion along the wash, a sandstone "float," and fossils in the limestone accent this path. Because the edge of the trail may be steep and dropoffs do exist, hikers should step carefully.

Oak Mountain State Park

Oak Mountain State Park, the largest in Alabama, stretches nearly 10,000 acres across Double Oak Mountain. Double Oak Mountain itself perches on the southernmost end of the Appalachian chain and has much the same terrain. The gently rolling hills, tall stands of timber, and clear lakes make this an ideal getaway for the afternoon or for several days. But its proximity to Alabama's largest city means that it gets a good deal of traffic, and on weekends in good weather, the park is especially crowded.

The park features an excellent golf course, a stocked lake for fishing, a marina with small boat rentals, stables, a demonstration farm, beaches, tennis courts, and even a motocross track. Camping, both primitive and recreational vehicle, is available for a fee, as are fully equipped cabins that will sleep eight. Oak Mountain State Park has recently become a popular destination for mountain bikers who also use one of the hiking trails.

The nature center resides in the park headquarters in

WEST CENTRAL ALABAMA

123

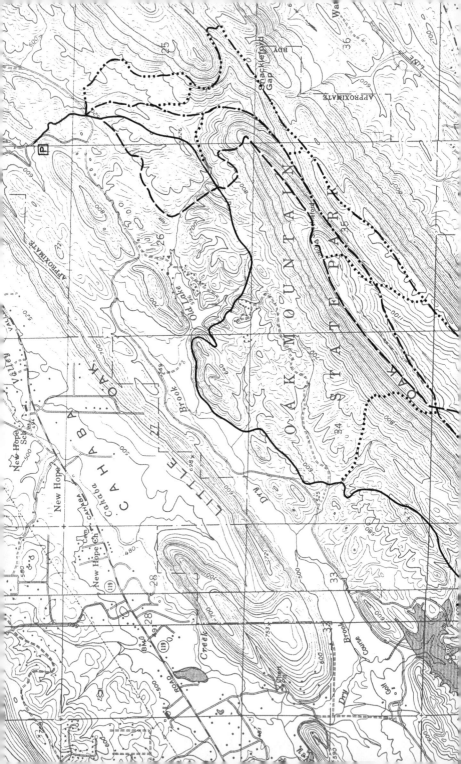

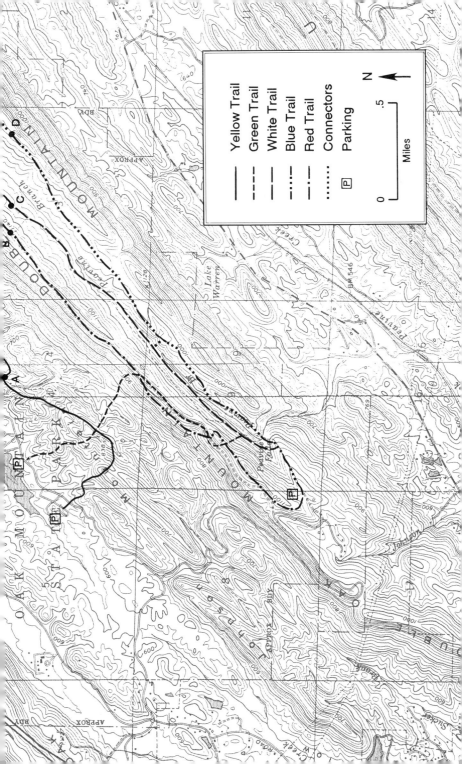

the day-use area and presents displays and programs on the flora and fauna of Oak Mountain State Park. Two short interpretive nature trails also originate across the road from the park headquarters. One, an elevated walkway called the Treetop Nature Trail, gives visitors a look at seldom-seen owls and hawks, permanently injured birds that have been given a home in the park through the auspices of the Wildlife Rescue Service. The nearby Buckeye Nature Trail, another easy, self-guiding walk, passes through some of the park's hardwood trees with their accompanying identification signs.

Plant and animal life differ little from one trail to the next because of the trails' proximity to one another. Dogwoods, hydrangeas, and wildflowers color the spring and summer months, and sweet gum, poplar, oak, sassafras, and hickory trees provide contrast to stately pines in autumn.

The 42 miles of trails here are all well marked and mostly moderate in degree of difficulty, depending on the direction traveled. The trails are much easier, of course, hiked from higher elevation to lower elevation. The distances for the trails in Oak Mountain State Park are given one-way, and the paths are generally described from the highest points to the lowest. Since these trails are well interconnected, a loop of almost any length is possible. Overnight camping is allowed along the trails, but hikers should use established locations and fire rings to lessen the impact of the campsites. Water is sometimes scarce along the trail, so hikers are advised to carry their own and to treat any that is taken, even from supposedly safe sources. The park, located 15 miles south of Birmingham off Interstate 65, is open from 7 A.M. to 9 P.M. daily, with a small fee for admission.

Topos: Chelsea, Helena 1:24,000

Yellow Trail

Length: 8 miles

Description: The longest trail in the park, Yellow Trail starts across the road from the day-use picnic area parking lot and ascends the heavily wooded hillside of Johnson Mountain. The trail soon turns north and snakes through large hickories and oaks for 2 miles before intersecting with the Yellow/White Connector, which joins Yellow Trail to White Trail. The trail descends toward Tranquility Lake, and skirts the shoreline for 0.5 mile. One mile later, it intersects with White Trail and the Yellow/Red Connector, which joins Yellow Trail with Red Trail. Yellow Trail passes through the north trailhead for Red and Blue trails and continues on to conclude at the country store. This trail too ranks as a moderate hike.

Green Trail

Length: 1.9 miles
Description: Green Trail, the shortest and steepest in the park, begins across the road from the park headquarters. The trail climbs the side of Johnson Mountain, intersecting with Yellow Trail and joining Red Trail for a short distance. After paralleling Red Trail for 0.5 mile, the pathway ascends steeply to meet White Trail and conclude at Peavine Falls. This trail should be considered difficult, owing to the steepness of the terrain.

White Trail

Length: 6.4 miles
Description: White Trail starts at the Peavine Falls parking lot and travels toward the falls, turning north along with Green Trail for a short distance. After passing the Blue/White Connector, which joins White Trail with Blue Trail, the pathway follows the ridgeline of Double Oak Mountain along an old jeep track. The pathway intersects Red Trail at the 2.5-mile point and continues to mount toward Shackleford Point, the park's highest point at 1,260 feet. The Orange Connector, located near the point, joins White Trail with Red and Blue trails. After passing the point, the pathway drops steeply within the next mile, crossing Yellow Trail and turning north again to end at the north trailhead along the park service road.

Blue Trail

Length: 6.7 miles
Description: Blue Trail, the most popular with backpackers, offers the best views of Double Oak Mountain and rural Shelby County. This moderate trail begins at the

WEST CENTRAL ALABAMA

Peavine Falls parking lot and travels north along Peavine Branch. At the 1-mile point, Blue Trail passes the White/Blue Connector, which joins White Trail to Blue Trail, and continues along the top of the ridge. Rocky outcroppings along the way offer many opportunities to stop and enjoy the panorama.

After passing the Orange Connector, which joins Blue Trail with both White and Red trails, the path begins to descend slightly. At mile 5 and mile 6, it passes the Red/Blue Connector, which joins Red Trail to Blue Trail. The path soon drops steadily off the hillside to end at the north trailhead along the park service road.

Red Trail

Length: 5.7 miles

Description: Red Trail begins near the Peavine Falls parking lot. This trail drops down the side of the hill for a short distance and parallels the ridgeline for much of its length. Into the trail 0.5 mile, it intersects with Green Trail and coincides with it for a short distance. The pathway keeps to a jeep track for the next 1.5 miles, before connecting with White Trail. Crossing the Orange Connector, which joins Blue Trail on the south to White Trail on the north, the trail begins to descend slightly. Red Trail connects twice in the next 2 miles, along the Red/Blue Connector, with Blue Trail before dropping finally to end at the north trailhead on the park service road. This, the most popular trail in the park, is a moderate hike over rolling terrain. This is the park's mountain biking trail as well, so hikers should watch for the extra traffic.

Rickwood Caverns State Park

Rickwood Caverns State Park holds the distinction of being the only caving park in the Alabama state park system. These 200-million-year-old caves are still considered active, living formations where water droplets form stalactites and stalagmites and flow into colorful shapes. Blind cave fish and bits of shell and marine fossils attest to the fact that this area was once an ocean bed. A camera figures as a valuable piece of equipment for this trip, as do

WEST CENTRAL
ALABAMA

128

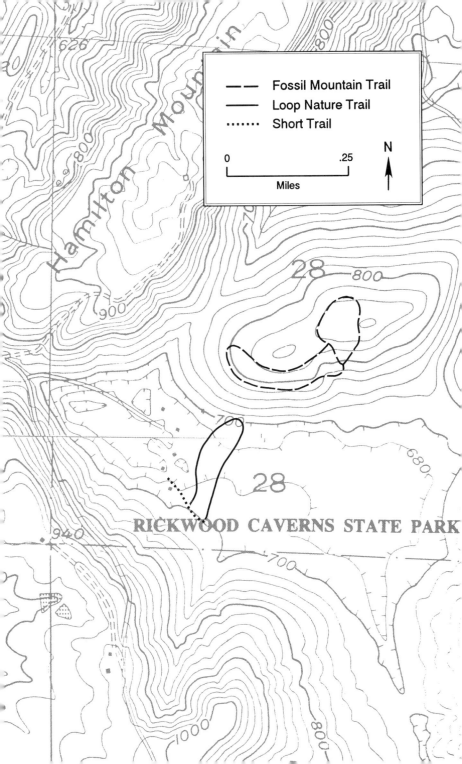

good walking shoes, for the rockiness of the terrain in some places makes careful footwork a necessity.

The mile-long cavern trail is open daily, 10 A.M. to 6 P.M., from Memorial Day to Labor Day and on weekends in the spring and fall but is closed November through February. Fees are charged for cave entrance, camping, and several of the entertainment facilities, though no fees are required for the hiking trails or the picnic area. Rickwood Caverns State Park is located off Interstate 65, north of Warrior, at exit 284 west.

Topos: Blount Springs, Warrior 1:24,000

Fossil Mountain Trail

Length: 1.3 miles

Description: This loop, the longest and the most interesting in the park, is considered a moderate hike because of the elevation gain and the boulder scrambling that must be done. The trail begins at the northwest end of the main parking area, behind the carpet golf course, where a sign directs the hiker to take the pathway to the right (northeast). Infrequent orange markers blaze trees and rocks as the pathway mounts among huge boulders and pines. The trail splits 0.25 mile up the hill, and the walker can continue in a straight line to an upper loop or turn left (west) to finish the lower loop. The upper loop is less obvious, as it climbs to the top of the hill for 0.25 mile and then drops and returns to the lower loop. The lower loop turns west and clings to the brow of the hill for a short distance, until it too drops down the hillside and returns to the starting point.

Loop Nature Trail

Length: 0.75 mile

Description: This self-guiding nature trail begins at the "Hiking Only" sign at the northeast corner of the parking lot and takes an easy stroll through pines, tulip poplars, and oaks. With yellow metallic tree markers, the loop is easily followed, although it can be confused with several dim traces that intersect in places with the main trail. The only hazards along the trail are the frequent sinkholes that are part of the cave system here. Hikers should not stray off the trail and should keep a close watch on small children. The loop connects, at both the main parking lot and the back of the picnic area, with Short Trail.

Short Trail

Length: 0.25 mile
Description: Short Trail, with yellow and red metallic tree markers, stands as a connector for the picnic area and Loop Nature Trail. The wide, almost flat, easily walked path begins at the south corner of the parking lot near the "Hiking Only" sign and joins Loop Nature Trail.

Tannehill Historical State Park

Tannehill Historical State Park is one of the newest and most unusual members of Alabama's state park system. The park is constructed around the ruins of the pre–Civil War Tannehill Furnaces and a multitude of historical reconstructions based on life in the mid-1800s. Pioneer cabins, a blacksmith shop, a gristmill, assorted antique farm machinery, craft cabins, and a museum with displays of furnace operation and community life provide a look into the birth of Birmingham's iron industry.

Plant life here is probably much the same as it was when the furnace was in use on the old Tannehill Plantation. Indian cucumber, Solomon's seal, wild roses, sweet cicely, and spiderwort line the trails, while a canopy of serviceberry, sweet gum, and oak trees provide shade.

The park has recreational vehicle and primitive campsites, a restaurant and snack shop, craft shops, picnic tables and pavilions, and playgrounds. The trails are short and easily walked and are for day hiking only. The well-marked trails and historical sites along them make the park an easy and enjoyable walking experience. Many of the trails interconnect, so an entire day can be spent with very little backtracking.

The park provides wheelchair accessibility for most of the visitor facilities, and a few of the trails may be wide and

WEST CENTRAL ALABAMA

131

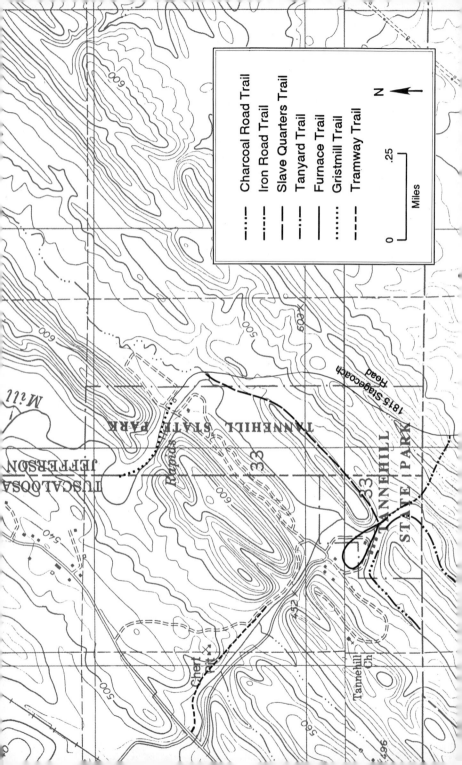

Legend

	Charcoal Road Trail
	Iron Road Trail
	Slave Quarters Trail
	Tanyard Trail
	Furnace Trail
	Gristmill Trail
	Tramway Trail

N

0   .25

Miles

TANNEHILL STATE PARK

TUSCALOOSA
JEFFERSON

1815 Stagecoach Road

TANNEHILL
STATE PARK

Tannehill
Ch

Chert
Pit

Roads

level enough for wheelchair access. At this writing, plans are being made for an additional 25-mile trail from Tannehill to the Brierfield state historic sites.

There is a small entrance fee to the park and a fee for camping. Tannehill Historical State Park is open daily from 7:00 A.M. to sunset. The park is located on Eastern Valley Road at the Bucksville exit off I-20/59, southwest of Birmingham.

Topos: Halfmile Shoals, McCalla 1:24,000

Charcoal Road Trail

Length: 0.7 mile

Description: This is a short, easy walk near Price Branch, originally where bushels of charcoal were carried to the Tannehill furnaces. The trail begins near the schoolhouse and follows the branch westward past the quarry and the drill rocks. The trail ends near the charcoal pits. Notice the drill holes in the sandstone where huge blocks were quarried to build the furnaces.

Iron Road Trail

Length: 2.5 miles

Description: The Iron Road Trail is so named because iron ingots from the Tannehill ironworks were shipped along this road by oxcart to the railroad at Montevallo. The trail starts near the beginning of the Slave Quarters Trail and moves south to cross into Bibb County and climb Double Team Hill. At the one-mile point, a side path takes the hiker to Oglesby Orchard. For the next mile the route is a gentle up-and-down walk, never far from the sound of Roupes Creek, until another side pathway leads one to the old Oglesby House site.

The trail ends at the interment site for many of the slaves who labored at the foundry and ironworks. The cemetery is estimated to hold three to four hundred graves.

Slave Quarters Trail

Length: 1.7 miles

Description: This wide, easy walkway is the main

road that Union troops used to attack the ironworks. The trail begins at the Slave Quarters Trail signpost near the bridge on the Roupes Creek. The trail passes the Grandfather Tree and then crosses a small bridge over a spring to join the old main road.

For the next mile this original roadbed passes the wagon-shop ruins, the remains of the Government House, and the old slave quarters, nearly all of which were burned as the Union soldiers raced to destroy the ironworks.

Tanyard Trail

Length: .08 mile
Description: This short walkway begins near the foundry and is a one-way stroll past the old tanning works, with some of the trees that characterize this area of Alabama. Look for beech trees, shagbark hickory trees, and sweet gums. This trail saw the hauling of much of the charcoal used in the ironwork foundry.

Furnace Trail

Length: 1.1 miles
Description: This easy trail begins near the park museum with a sign to mark its starting point and quickly crosses a small creek called Price Branch. Walkers can envision daily life in the mid-1800s while passing the four cabins along the first quarter-mile of this trail.

The trail soon passes the quarry site and enters the restored ironworks area that was in operation until destroyed in a Union attack on March 31, 1865. After passing the blower house and forge, the trail loops past the foundry to follow the tramway, past the drill rocks area and back to its beginning.

Gristmill Trail

Length: 0.7 mile
Description: The Gristmill Trail parallels Cooley Creek and allows the walker to view Hall's Mill. The trail starts near the bridge at the Mill site and ends at the boundary fence at the park. Look for wild roses near the fence and sweet cicely along the trail.

Tramway Trail

Length: 0.8 mile

Description: The Tramway Trail starts on the rock dam beside the park's Furnace Master Restaurant. The trail traces the route of the tramway where oxcarts hauled ore from the mines to the ironworks. After crossing the dam the route travels northwest, paralleling the park's entrance road, and ends near the site of the first gristmill at Tannehill and the site of an old dam that serviced the mill.

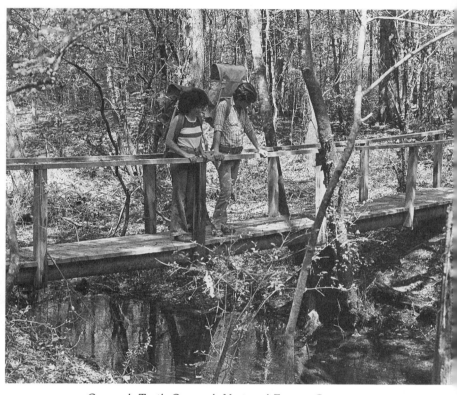

Conecuh Trail, Conecuh National Forest, Covington County (Photograph by Joy Patty, Courtesy the U.S. Department of Agriculture, Forest Service)

Trails in South Alabama

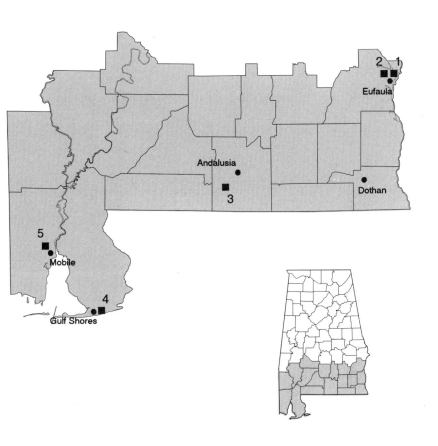

1. Eufaula National Wildlife Refuge
2. Lakepoint Resort State Park
3. Conecuh National Forest
4. Gulf State Park
5. Chickasabogue Park

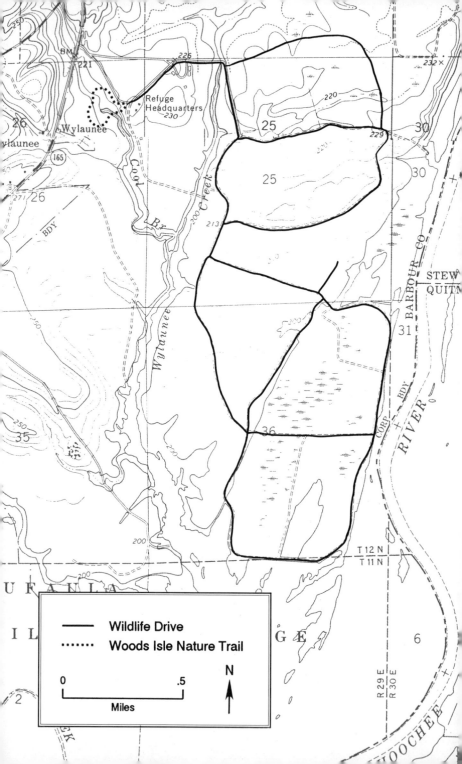

Eufaula National Wildlife Refuge

Eufaula National Wildlife Refuge was established in 1964 in a cooperative effort between the U.S. Fish and Wildlife Service and the U.S. Army Corps of Engineers. The refuge encompasses over 11,000 acres of improved habitat and feeding areas for wildlife and waterfowl. Creatures of the woodland, such as raccoons, deer, opossums, foxes, and squirrels, abound year-round, while winter visitors include up to 16 different species of ducks and 4 types of geese.

Woods Isle Nature Trail and Wildlife Drive, both self-guiding and well marked, are open during daylight hours, with no fees for day use. Restrooms, drinking water, and maps of the area are available at the refuge office from 7:30 A.M. to 4 P.M. weekdays and Saturdays.

Fishing and hunting, under special conditions, are permitted, and public boat launches are located throughout the refuge. Lakepoint Resort State Park lies nearby and offers full facilities for campers and a marina. Eufaula National Wildlife Refuge is located 7 miles north of the city of Eufaula on U.S. 431 and 2 miles northeast on Alabama 165.

Topos: Georgetown, Georgia-Alabama; Twin Springs, Georgia-Alabama 1:24,000

Wildlife Drive

Length: 5 miles

Description: Those who want a longer trip and a much closer look at the residents of the refuge should hike all or a portion of Wildlife Drive. The 5-mile looping road makes the walking easy and takes the hiker through all the different habitat sites and around the various impoundments, and without a noisy automobile, the animals and birds don't seem to mind the intrusion. In one 2-hour period, the author rubbed shoulders with the refuge's resident flock of Canada geese, a flock of wild turkeys, a mass of semitame rabbits, and an alligator whose tameness we did not care to investigate. The auto loop was a very pleasurable alternative to the nature trail, well worth spending a day touring. Late afternoon, when most of the birds settle down to roost, the hiker is most likely to see the

SOUTH ALABAMA

139

greatest variety in waterfowl, as well as animals. Spring and autumn are the most pleasant times of the year to visit.

Woods Isle Nature Trail

Length: 0.5 mile

Description: This loop begins 50 yards west of the refuge office and wanders in several smaller loops through this marshy wooded area. Benches are provided for those wishing to stop and watch the myriad of birds here, and signs are posted along the trail to identify trees, such as post and laurel oaks, magnolias, maples, and loblolly pines. Plants of all types may be seen in natural settings, including muscadine vines and various ferns. The trail crosses a small stream at one point, and a wooden bridge serves as another convenient observation point for wildlife.

Lakepoint Resort State Park

Lakepoint Resort State Park is one of Alabama's splendid park resorts, with a lodge, campgrounds, marina, cabins, and, apparently as an afterthought, trails. Situated on the shoreline of Walter F. George Reservoir, more familiarly known as Lake Eufaula, this area is famous for bass fishing and boating and is geared more to campers rather than hikers, offering primitive camping as well as a full-service recreational vehicle campground, a large picnic area, a golf course, tennis courts, and a beach area. No fees are levied for day use and only small fees for camping and some concessions, such as boat rentals. The trails here are easy and short with no particular hazards.

The main facilities of Lakepoint Resort State Park, on U.S. 431 just 7 miles north of Eufaula, are situated at the confluence of Cowikee Creek and the 46,000-acre lake formed by a dammed-up stretch of the Chattahoochee River. The nearby Eufaula Wildlife Refuge holds an enormous draw for wildlife of all sorts and waterfowl for most of the year.

Topos: Eufaula North, Georgetown, Georgia-Alabama 1:24,000

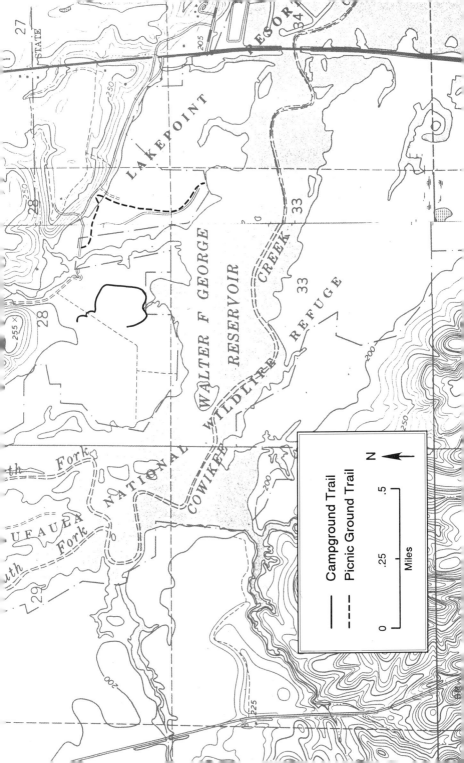

Campground Trail

Length: 1.5 miles

Description: The trail, a clear-cut road that runs behind the Deer Court vehicle camping area, starts near the camp store, where parking is available. No elevation gain or loss exists, nor do other problems for walkers, with the exception of the occasional snake and poison ivy. Strollers will notice a large variety of birds, as well as pines, dogwoods, and oaks. The trail circles the Deer Court campground and ends on the south side of the area. Intermittent brown wooden fences delineate entrances to the trail at several locations, including the main service road.

Picnic Ground Trail

Length: 0.5 mile

Description: This trail, an easy stroll, starts at the main service road just west of the entrance to the picnic area, parallels the service road through a wooded lane, and then veers south to end at the lakefront.

Conecuh National Forest

The 80,000-acre Conecuh National Forest has a system of four trails with a combined length of over 20 miles. And because of its southernmost location, the Conecuh is a perfect winter hiking destination for those who prefer milder conditions and fewer insects but still wish to get into the outdoors. The abundance of trailside water (which should be purified for use), the lack of any significant grade, and a surface of packed sand and pine needles make the hiking easy for almost anyone. The trails are blazed with light gray metal diamonds on trees, and wooden footbridges over wet areas are provided where needed. Forest service (FS) roads also may be hiked and used for access to portions of the trails, although some are closed to vehicular traffic from March 10 to October 15. Photographers will enjoy the abundant variety of wildlife and the picturesque qualities of the many cypress ponds along the trail.

SOUTH ALABAMA

Primitive camping is permitted on the trail, with the exception of hunting season (mid-November to late April), which, unfortunately, is the most attractive time in the Conecuh. Special permits to camp during this period may be obtained from the local district ranger in Andalusia. Camping is available at the Blue Pond and Open Pond recreation areas, as are potable water, restroom facilities, picnic sites, unsupervised swimming, and fishing. The Open Pond Recreation Area is the largest and is open year-round. One caution to hikers involves the large number of alligators (estimated at over 450) in the areas around the ponds. Alligators can be dangerous, and those traveling near wet areas and wading or swimming in the ponds themselves (not recommended) should take care not to aggravate this particular local population.

The Conecuh National Forest resides in Covington and Escambia counties, with the best access to camping and the trail system at the Open Pond Recreation Area off Alabama (AL) 137, 17 miles south of Andalusia.

Topos: Carolina, Wing 1:24,000

Conecuh Trail

Length: 24 miles

Description: Conecuh Trail, the longest in the national forest, includes portions of the other pathways. One starting point for Conecuh Trail is at the Open Pond Recreation Area, which also offers the most secure parking for automobiles. The trail begins across the road from the parking area and travels through a wooded area toward Buck Pond, which, along with nearby Ditch Pond, Open Pond, and Five Runs Creek, offers the best bass and bream fishing on this particular section of the trail. After passing Buck Pond, the path crosses a small stream and meanders through a succession of pine ridges and hardwood bottoms to intersect FS 348A and FS 337. The trail parallels the course of Five Runs Creek for 0.25 mile, passing Blue Spring, a large freshwater spring and popular summer swimming hole. A parking area is located at Blue Spring, with access to the area via forest service roads. Passing the parking area, the trail turns west back toward the ponds, crossing FS 337, FS 348A, and FS 348. After crossing FS 348 at 0.5 mile, the trail divides, the Conecuh

SOUTH
ALABAMA

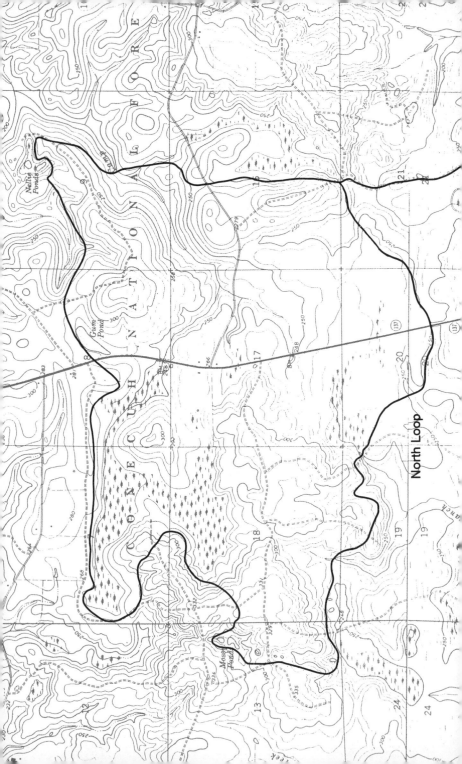

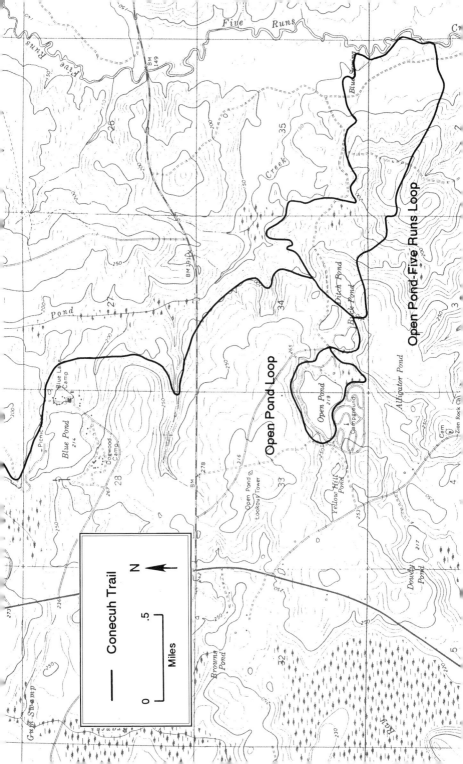

Trail going north and the Open Pond–Five Runs Loop turning south.

Close to where the trail turns north, an offshoot of the path takes the hiker to a natural spring, a good place for a break and perhaps lunch. The trail crosses County 24, where another parking area is provided, and a mile farther enters the Blue Pond Recreation Area, which has facilities for camping and is another good fishing spot. A mile north from Blue Pond, the trail branches to form the 10.5-mile North Loop and intersects FS 335.

Continuing northward for 2 miles on the somewhat overgrown pathway will bring the hiker to the two Nellie Ponds and several crossings of FS 325. Another parking area and access point is located a mile past the Nellie Ponds at the trail's intersection with AL 137. The trail traverses the highway and continues west, paralleling FS 330 and heading for the Mossy Ponds area. These small cypress ponds represent some of the prettiest in the forest, and the lack of undergrowth and openness of the forest make this area a pleasure to hike. This end of the trail also has the highest elevations in the Conecuh, often reaching 300 feet above sea level. The trail moves through the shelter of tall pines, frequently intersecting service roads, for approximately 3 miles, until it once again crosses AL 137 and another small parking area. One mile past the parking area, the trail completes the loop and turns south along the same pathway back past Blue Pond toward Open Pond and the original parking location.

Open Pond Loop

Length: 1.5 miles

Description: Open Pond Loop, also known as Lake Shore Trail, takes an easy hike around one of the most popular facilities in the Conecuh National Forest. The trail begins at the hiking sign on the service road into the Open Pond Recreation Area. The pathway leads north up the side of the hill into the woods that surround the pond. Although easily hiked, the path is overgrown in some places and blurred by the cutting of right-of-way for utility poles. The trail rambles through the woods for 0.5 mile, until it drops off the hill to traverse the campground road and follow the shoreline for another 0.5 mile. The trail finally passes the campground and skirts a marshy depression to join the Open Pond–Five Runs Loop and return to the service road.

Open Pond–Five Runs Loop

Length: 5 miles
Description: This trail starts at a hiking sign just off the picnic area service road, passes Buck Pond, and then turns south to travel through the woods (see also Conecuh Trail), crossing a small stream and two forest service roads. After approximately 2 miles, the pathway nears Five Runs Creek and parallels its course for 0.5 mile to Blue Spring, a large freshwater spring that makes a fine rest or lunch stop. After leaving the spring, it passes the Blue Spring parking area, and the hiker can stroll under a canopy of large pines and through fields of ferns, until the trail once again begins to climb low ridges and enter denser undergrowth. Over the next 2 miles, the trail intersects FS 337, FS 348A, and FS 348 and then passes the northward turnoff to Conecuh Trail. To complete the loop, the trail turns south and passes Ditch and Buck ponds and reenters the Open Pond Recreation Area along the same route as its beginning.

North Loop

Length: 10.5 miles
Description: North Loop Trail is bisected by AL 137 and has a parking location at either point for the purposes of starting this trail (see also Conecuh Trail). Beginning at the north parking lot and traveling west, the trail heads toward the Mossy Ponds area, paralleling FS 330 through tall pines and magnolias for approximately 2.5 miles. The trail then crosses FS 350C and FS 350E before circling the ponds and turning south. On the southern portion of the loop, the trail passes several small ponds and intersects FS 329, FS 330F, and FS 355.

One mile past the trail's southern crossing of AL 137, the trail meets the Blue Pond entrance to North Loop at FS 335, and hikers who prefer a more secure parking area and camping facilities may choose to walk in from this point. The trek from Blue Pond is about 1 mile and would add a total of 2 miles to the length of the loop if hiked from this direction. From this point, it is a 2-mile walk to Nellie Ponds, with the only problem being trail overgrowth, and then a 1-mile walk to Gum Pond and the completion of the loop at the parking area at AL 137.

Gulf State Park

Considered the showcase of Alabama's magnificent park resort system, Gulf State Park perches on some of the most beautiful beachfront on the Gulf of Mexico. This resort has not only the standard vacation beach attractions but also facilities for meetings and conventions, with a gulfside restaurant and cocktail lounge. And in addition to the hotel facilities, cabins and recreational vehicle and tent camping spaces are available. Visitors can fish from the pier, which extends 800 feet into the gulf, or in either of the two freshwater lakes, or they can play golf on an 18-hole course.

The Creek Indians, who were probably the first to see these trails, would no doubt be amazed at what has been done to this stretch of coastline, although still to be found here are the pines, magnolias, and palmettos and the alligators and other animal life that have long characterized marshlands and coastal terrain. The trails, almost always level and well marked, are sandy, so good shoes are advisable. At certain times of the year, snakes and insects are a problem as well—another good reason for stout shoes. Alligators are residents of the park, and hikers can almost always spot one or more, usually in the water along the Middle Lake Trail. Alligators will eat almost anything, but they are dangerous wild animals, and visitors should refrain from feeding them. Rangers also advise that careless dogs are a favorite food of the alligators, so precautions should be taken with pets.

Gulf State Park, located near Gulf Shores off Alabama 182, is open year-round, and visitors are welcome in daylight hours. A fee is charged for day use at the lake area but none for the beach area. Trail maps and information sheets are available at the campground registration building and at the ranger's station.

Topo: Gulf Shores 1:24,000

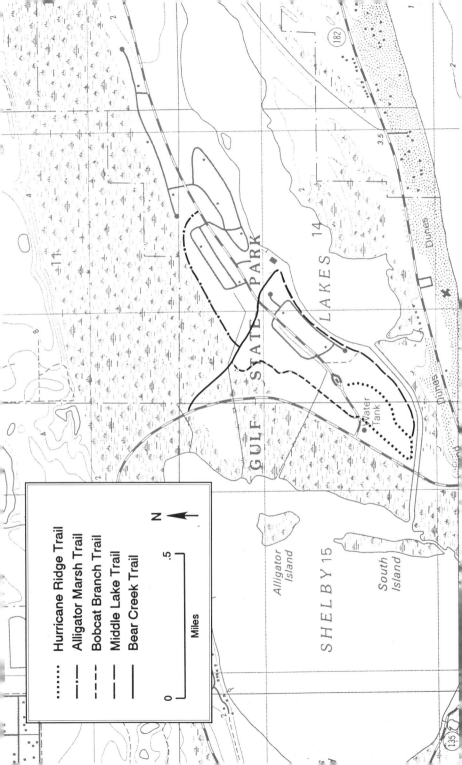

Legend

...... Hurricane Ridge Trail
–·–· Alligator Marsh Trail
– – – Bobcat Branch Trail
——— Middle Lake Trail
——— Bear Creek Trail

N

Miles
0   .5

GULF STATE PARK

LAKES 14

Dunes

Dunes

Water
Tank

SHELBY 15

Alligator
Island

South
Island

182

135

Hurricane Ridge Trail

Length: 0.7 mile

Description: Hurricane Ridge Trail, also known as the Nature Discovery Trail, begins at the camper check-in station. The trail itself has a sand base, so walking can be tedious if that is not the hiker's favorite surface. But the sand also easily shows the tracks of the vast number of animals that inhabit this area, and fox and raccoon tracks are especially common when the muscadine grapes are plentiful. The trail is easily traveled, so it is possible to look around and notice the remnants of the damage done by Hurricane Frederick in September of 1979. The 130-mph winds battered and uprooted thousands of trees along this part of the gulf. Many of these dead trees are still standing, however, and these provide homes for numerous insects, as well as the woodpeckers who feast on them. Saw palmettos with their palmlike leaves and large roots growing above the soil are especially noticeable, as are the live oak trees that are home to the park's many squirrels. The trail loops and then dead ends at the main road into the camping area.

Alligator Marsh Trail

Length: 0.7 mile

Description: This trail starts near the Bear Creek crossing on Bear Creek Trail and ends at the campground service road. Currently under construction, this trail is not marked after the entrance and traverses a marshy area much favored by snakes. Travel is not advised for any but the most adventurous souls.

Bobcat Branch Trail

Length: 0.8 mile

Description: Bobcat Branch Trail starts across the campground service road from Hurricane Ridge Trail and takes an easy stroll through saw palmettos, live oaks, and blackberry brambles. Bordering the trail in many areas is the saw grass that provides cover for marsh rabbits, distinguishable from cottontails by their darker color and lack of a white tail. Bobcat Branch Trail ends at the

SOUTH
ALABAMA

150

intersection with Bear Creek Trail near the bridge crossing.

Middle Lake Trail

Length: 1.5 miles

Description: Middle Lake Trail begins at the nature center and follows the canal that connects Middle Lake to Lake Shelby. This is the best area to observe the alligators that inhabit the park. They are very good at hiding in the long grass at the water's edge along the canal, so sometimes only eyes and nose are all that can be seen. The trail is an easy, relatively flat walk and ends at its intersection with Hurricane Ridge Trail.

Bear Creek Trail

Length: 0.8 mile

Description: Bear Creek Trail has the easiest access in the park and is suitable even for handicapped traffic, since it is an old paved road. The trail starts at the nature center and moves through the campground, traversing the access road and then joining the pavement. At approximately the halfway mark, the road crosses a small stream, Bear Creek, where fanciers of wild medicinal plants will note arrowhead, pickerelweed, and water lilies. The trail ends at County 2, where the hiker can retrace his steps or return to camp on the road. The trail also intersects Bobcat Branch Trail and Alligator Marsh Trail near the stream crossing.

Chickasabogue Park

Situated in the heart of urban Mobile County, Chickasabogue Park in Prichard is a 1,050-acre park that may be unfamiliar to even local residents. The area is covered in hardwoods, swampland, and pockets of wilderness, with deer, foxes, opossums, egrets, and alligators as frequent visitors. The park is even more unusual in that it provides wilderness canoe trails and nature trails in the same facility. Chickasabogue Park is named for the creek that forms one of its boundaries and for the adjacent

SOUTH
ALABAMA

151

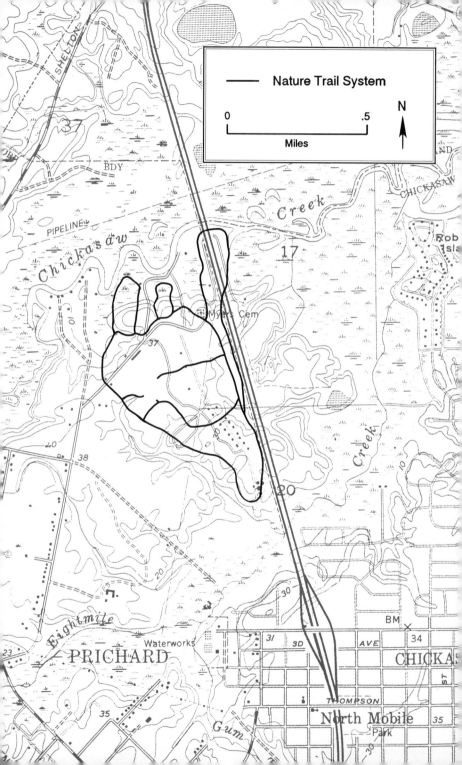

Nature Trail System

0 5
Miles
N

swamp, which has seen its share of Chickasaw Indian skirmishes, a Civil War battle, and the march of Andrew Jackson to the Battle of New Orleans.

The park is open seven days a week from 7 A.M. to sundown and has a small admission fee. Camping facilities with hookups, fishing and beach areas, and canoe rentals are available. Information sheets and trail maps can be picked up at the museum and information center at the entrance to the park.

To get to the park, follow Interstate 65 (local), take the U.S. 45 West exit (St. Stephens Road), turn right (north) on Alabama 213, take the first right turn after the railroad tracks (Culvert Street), then left on Adcock Road to the park entrance. For more information, contact Chickasabogue Park, 760 Adcock Road, Prichard, Alabama 36613.

Topo: Chickasaw 1:24,000

Nature Trail System

Length: Approximately 10 miles

Description: Chickasabogue Park features an interconnecting network of 10 footpaths and trails that showcases the variety of flora and fauna in this area. The Nature Trail is a 0.7-mile loop off the park service road, the entrance to which is marked by signs. Look for cypress, magnolia, and cedar trees, as well as huge wild azaleas along this trail. Another spot of note is the cemetery of the Meyers family, owners of a pre–Civil War plantation that was located on the current park site. The trails are easy to walk, although overgrown in places. Late spring and summer (during Mobile's "Festival of Humidity") may not be the ideal time to take in the sights of the park, since the mosquitoes and gnats have voracious appetites.

Suggested Readings

Dean, Blanche E., Amy Mason, and Joab L. Thomas. *Wildflowers of Alabama and Adjoining States.* Tuscaloosa: University of Alabama Press, 1973.

Doan, Marilyn. *Hiking Light.* Magnolia, Mass.: Peter Smith, 1983.

Fletcher, Colin. *The Complete Walker III.* 3d ed. New York: Alfred A. Knopf, 1984.

Gibbons, Whit, Robert R. Haynes, and Joab L. Thomas. *Poisonous Plants and Venomous Animals of Alabama and Adjoining States.* Tuscaloosa: University of Alabama Press, 1990.

Hart, John. *Walking Softly in the Wilderness: The Sierra Club Guide to Backpacking.* Rev. ed. San Francisco: Sierra Club, 1984.

Manning, Harvey. *Backpacking: One Step at a Time, New 1980's Edition.* 3d ed. New York: Random House, 1980.

Mount, Robert H. *Reptiles and Amphibians of Alabama.* Auburn, Ala.: Auburn University Agricultural Experiment Station, 1975; distributed by University of Alabama Press.

Peters, Edward, ed. *Mountaineering: The Freedom of the Hills.* 4th ed. Seattle: Mountaineers, 1982.

Thurmond, John T., and Douglas E. Jones. *Fossil Vertebrates of Alabama.* Tuscaloosa: University of Alabama Press, 1981.

Winnett, Thomas, and Melaine Findling. *Backpacking Basics.* 3d ed. Berkeley: Wilderness Press, 1988.

Index of Trails

INDEX

OF TRAILS

About the Author

Pat Sharpe, having hiked over 95 percent of the trails in Alabama, began researching the trails for customers and friends while managing a trail shop in Montgomery. In addition to leading hiking and paddling trips for friends, Sharpe has been active in the Sierra Club and in wildflower groups. She now lives with her husband and a loaner cat in Biloxi, Mississippi.